Preventing

ALZHEIMER'S
AGGRESSION

| SUPPORTIVE |

| THERAPY |

| IN ACTION |

BY LEN FABIANO

B O O K   T W O

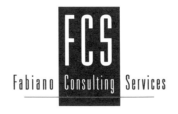

COPYRIGHT 1996

ISBN #0-9695584-9-X

FCS Publications
Fabiano Consulting Services Inc.

P.O. Box 777
Edgewater, Florida
32132

P.O. Box 1300
Seagrave, Ontario
L0C 1G0

FCS provides a wide range of services to the health care industry including; in-house seminars, consultation, publications and audio-visual material.

For further information and a free catalogue, contact:

Mr. Len Fabiano
FCS President
(800)387-8143

DEDICATED TO:

Robbie Sprules

Valued friend and associate.

Your creativity and imagination has provided the direction. Your encouragement and support has provided the motivation.

Acknowledgments

To the dedicated caregivers who have shown me the skills and to the mentally impaired who have led the way.

To Cheryl Graham who has become a valuable asset to my work and our organization. To Joan Graham for the value of her experience. A special thank you to Ron Martyn, Kim Blakely and Ron Douglas, whose friendship, support and assistance is greatly appreciated

To my family - my wife Linda, my son Daniel and my daughter Kimberly - for their support through <u>one more book</u>. I could never accomplish the things I do without your encouragement.

Len

ABOUT THE AUTHOR

MR. LEN FABIANO has trained over 180,000 people nationwide on a variety of topics concerning care of the elderly and long term care, and worked with scores of health care facilities and organizations to enhance their efficiency and effectiveness. Author of _five popular texts_ on aging and long term care, he has become well known for his effective, practical approaches to dealing with highly complex issues. As a Gerontologist, Nurse and Counselor, Len's extensive experience in Long Term Care adds depth to his educational material and seminars. Len's sessions not only educate and entertain, but excite those who attend to become more effective at what they do and how they do it.

Mr. Fabiano is the founder and president of Fabiano Consulting Services. FCS has become a well recognized and dynamic corporation specializing in education and consulting services to health care organizations (with a focus on long term care). FCS publishes and distributes Mr. Fabiano's books worldwide, and produces his popular video series. FCS provides consulting services to help organizations improve staff/management relations and overall efficiency, and enhance direct care programs and environmental design. Len Fabiano's other texts include:

> _**Working With The Frail Elderly:**_ Beyond The Physical Disability (second edition)
>
> _**The Tactics Of Supportive Therapy:**_ A Comprehensive Intervention Program on Caring for the Alzheimer's Victim (second edition)
>
> _**Mother I'm Doing The Best I Can:**_ Families of Aged Parents during Times of Loss and Crisis
>
> _**Getting Staff Excited:**_ The Role of the Nurse Manager (And Others Too) in Long Term Care (second edition)

CONTENTS

OPENING

I was asked to conduct a quick assessment of a unit housing the mentally impaired. Part way through the assessment, while talking to one of the staff, there was an explosion by the cupboards next to me. I looked at the cupboards and then on the floor. There was broken glass scattered everywhere. On the other side of me was a small mentally impaired lady saying repeatedly, "You want to hurt someone, you hurt me. Do you understand?" Apparently she had thrown a glass vase at me and missed. (Thank goodness her aim was bad.)

I asked a staff member to take her down the hall in hopes of distracting her from whatever my presence was initiating. The resident would have none of that. She insisted on staying, repeating her phrase, becoming increasingly more agitated. She followed me as I left the unit, having to be physically blocked from going through the secured doors after me. Apparently it took staff considerable time to settle her after I was gone.

Staff shared with me later that this lady may have been abused in the past. They felt that my beard was the trigger. Her linking me with that person in her past apparently sparked her aggression.

Caring for the Alzheimer's victim is probably the most demanded topic in the field of aging. There are tremendous amounts of new information generated yearly on this specialty. It is so complex that no one book ever seems adequate enough to cover all of the needs and interventions for this clientele. This is the reason for writing this text.

I have received continuous feedback that my text, <u>The Tactics of Supportive Therapy (Book One)</u> has been a highly successful resource in providing direction on caring for the mentally impaired elderly. Likewise, the concepts of *Supportive Therapy* have apparently helped caregivers to clarify the needs of the mentally impaired and provide a variety of practical and effective tools to perform quality care. However, it was not enough. The needs go beyond that one book.

Working with scores of mentally impaired clients, consulting with many organizations, counseling family members of Alzheimer's victims, training thousands of health care professionals over the years has uncovered two things - the vulnerability of this clientele and the frustration of the caregivers. The majority of caregivers, whether family or professional, demonstrated a constant desire to provide the greatest level of quality care possible, with considerable passion. Unfortunately they became frustrated when at times their efforts were met with continued resistance or even hostility on the part of their client.

Years ago, I was asked repeatedly to present an educational workshop on how to deal with Alzheimer's aggression. There seemed little basis for a seminar. Dealing with Alzheimer's aggression when it occurred only had a few interventions available - back off, sedate or restrain. None of these were entirely successful and some were even detrimental.

When examining the instances of Alzheimer's aggression, two re-occurring issues surfaced -

⇒ *this client possessed a unique vulnerability.*
⇒ *generally when aggression occurred it was the result of what was going on around or to the person.*

It finally became obvious. The focus was wrong - waiting until a mentally impaired client became aggressive was too late. The vast majority of aggressive outbursts with the Alzheimer's victim were *preventable*.

This led to the seminar Preventing Alzheimer's Aggression. Thousands of caregivers and family members have attended that session. It expanded the skills of some, corroborated the abilities of others and gave others a whole new view of this clientele. The response to the content of those sessions became the motivation for writing this text.

THIS IS BOOK TWO

This is not a repeat of my book the Tactics of Supportive Therapy (Book One). That text detailed the experiences of the mentally impaired and the concepts of *Supportive Therapy*. Of course in this work, it has been necessary to summarize and/or make reference to certain aspects of that text. However, Preventing Alzheimer's Aggression: Supportive Therapy in Action is *book two*. It takes that material and focuses it on aggressive behavior only.

An overview of this text is as follows. Chapter One of Preventing Alzheimer's Aggression discusses the experiences of being mentally impaired, the disease and the degree of vulnerability associated with the disease process. If you have read the text The Tactics of Supportive Therapy, it is important to read this chapter. Not only does it summarize some of the information presented in the earlier text, but it demonstrates how it specifically relates to aggressive behavior. If you have not read that text, you may want to refer to The Tactics of Supportive Therapy to expand on what is presented. The information from that text establishes the foundation to understanding and dealing with aggressive behavior of the mentally impaired elderly.

Chapter Two presents a detailed case that will demonstrate the needs of this clientele and what can lead to aggressive behavior. Chapter Three describes what is called the Aggressive Episode, the Chronic Aggressive Pattern and the Violent Episode.

Chapter Four details the *thirty-two causes of aggressive behavior*, and how the care conferencing assessment process called Care Analysis can be used. This chapter also examines aggression as it applies to the mentally impaired elderly, the difficulties aggressive behavior can create, and what can be expected.

The next three chapters focus on programming. Assessment tools are outlined in Chapter Five, programming options in Chapter Six and what is called the Controlling Approach in Chapter Seven. The final chapter provides the opportunity to assess the care environment within your setting, your personal abilities, and defines the challenges that this clientele presents.

THE CONTENT

This is not simply a "how to text" on dealing with *aggression*. The material discussed is very specific. It focuses on *Alzheimer's aggression* only. Some are surprised at the distinction, thinking that the concepts that apply to any aggressive behavior should be universal for all types of clients. In actual fact that is not the case. The mentally impaired demonstrate a dramatic difference based on the uniqueness of the disease process occurring, their symptomology and the resultant vulnerability.

These qualities create characteristics that must be reflected in the programming and intervention strategies employed. To scan this book and only look at the intervention strategies presented in the final chapters, will only have limited value. This is a progressive text. Each chapter builds on the last and sets the foundation for the next. Without understanding the relationship of the disease to the interventions, the strategies will not be totally successful. It is imperative that you work through each section of this book in order to gain the most from the material presented.

Likewise, this is not a passive text. You will not be allowed only to read. In all of my texts, I have employed a highly successful writing technique called *Guided Imagery*. This approach allows the reader to personalize the experience discussed. This style requires from you a commitment to be involved in order to participate in what you are about to read. Do not take the technique lightly. It is not a mere form of entertainment, but a valuable and powerful tool that will clarify what you read and increase your comprehension of the concepts presented.

The instructions for the process of Guided Imagery are as follows:

Your task is to read each scenario adding a slight twist. You will notice certain phrases are broken with a slash(/). The purpose of each slash is to have you pause; internalize what you have just read; form a mental image of what was described; and then move to the next statement. Take your time and work slowly through each one you encounter. In these exercises it is important that you *hear* yourself as you read, so that you can *see* the sequence of events, and *feel* the consequences as they apply to you.

Hear it, See it and Feel it.

LIMITATIONS

When writing a text like this, it is necessary to demonstrate points succinctly. When examples are presented in isolation, they do not always represent what an organization or caregiver is doing that is positive and effective. The case example in chapter two demonstrates this well. It is a dramatic depiction of what can cause aggressive behavior in the mentally impaired. Reading that case can create a misinterpretation of long term care in general. In actual fact, the facility identified provided excellent care to their cognitively well, physically disabled clients. Unfortunately, they were ill-equipped to care for the mentally impaired and the specific client discussed.

There is a significant polarization of long term care organizations within our industry. Some facilities and community based programs are impressive. They have been highly innovative and creative, working well with the mentally impaired. They have become the pace setters, the trend makers, developing new and innovative strategies on enhancing the quality of life for this clientele. Other organizations have successfully developed certain aspects of their care, but are still lacking in other areas to reach their full effectiveness. Still others have been delinquent in preparing for this clientele at all. Of course of the three groups, it is the latter two that best define the need, and the first two that have found many of the solutions.

In fact, what seems to contribute most to the incidence of aggressive behavior of the mentally impaired, is the circumstances that exist within some organizations.

- A client population that has changed from cognitively well to mentally impaired.
- Limited training in caring for the mentally impaired elderly.
- A lack of appropriate programming for this clientele.
- Employing intervention strategies that worked well with the cognitively well.
- An environmental design geared for the cognitively well.
- Minimal behavioral and functional assessment tools.
- Out-dated care routines.
- Limited empowering of staff.

Organizations that demonstrated any one or more of these issues seemed to experience an increased occurrence of aggressive behavior among their mentally impaired clients. Subsequently, as each of these issues were resolved, aggressive behavior of the mentally impaired decreased.

The mentally impaired are a highly unique clientele who require specialization in the care provided. Until recently, long term care has not had the urgency to move into this specialty with vigor and haste. There was not a sufficient need. Now as most organizations find their client population comprised primarily of the mentally impaired, the behavioral response of this clientele dictate that the organization's energies and resources be invested in this direction. Some organizations are already there, others are moving forward and still others have a long way to go.

THE MOTIVATION FOR THIS TEXT

This text introduces you to a term called the *Investigative Caregiver*. These are caregivers who are *proactive*, attempting to deal with the behavior before it occurs, rather than reactive, waiting for the behavior to occur.

The *investigative caregiver* knows that the low functioning mentally impaired do not have the ability to analyze their situation and articulate what they experience. Instead, they respond to things that distress them through their behavior.

The *investigative caregiver* looks for the clues and assembles a picture from the fragmented information about this person's past history, behavioral responses, vulnerability, symptoms, abilities and losses. Once the cues are interpreted, they usually point to a causative factor that justifies this individual's behavior. Once the cause is known, steps can then be taken to prevent the aggressive response from occurring again.

That is the major challenge in caring for this clientele. To be successful, you must be a detective or "investigator." You must have the understanding and skills that set you apart from the rest.

Let us begin the detective work.
The case is fascinating and complex.
The rewards are substantial.

Chapter One

ESTABLISHING THE FOUNDATION

There is a popular simulation entitled "Walk-A-Day-In-My-Shoes." It allows caregivers the opportunity to simulate a mock disability in order to understand first hand what it may be like to be physically disabled. During this exercise, some participants will have their right arm tied to their body and right leg tied to the leg of their chair to simulate a stroke, others will have their fingers taped together to simulate arthritis, and still others will have their eyes covered to simulate blindness, and so on. After they are readied, they will be asked to perform a normal daily task such as eating a meal.

Those who have experienced such a simulation usually report a dramatic affect - they more closely experience and feel the frustrations and challenges of what it may mean to be disabled. It is a very effective technique that helps caregivers gain further insight into why some disabled older people may withdraw and others become aggressive under such circumstances.

Unfortunately there is no exercise that will simulate mental impairment as well as "Walk-A-Day-In-My-Shoes" simulates physical disability. Understanding how a mentally impaired client may view his world is no easy task. The best that can be done is to compare this experience to something that may be common to many of us.

Imagine:

> You are hiking or sight seeing in the woods/
> After a short while
> You become lost/
> How would you feel once you realized that you were lost?

You probably would encounter a twinge of anxiety. At this point you would probably be confident that the next turn would provide you with a way out.

> How would you feel 3 hours and 55 minutes later?
> Five minutes before you find your way out?

For most, that initial anxiety would easily turn into panic. When panic ensues, you could find yourself wandering around in circles, passing the same tree time and time again without even noticing it. The more intense the panic, the less one's ability to think clearly and problem solve. The experience for most would be quite frightening and distressing.

> During the entire time that you are lost
> Why would you keep walking?
> What would you be looking for?

A person who is lost will constantly walk in an attempt to find something familiar - a rock, trail, stream, etc. Anything that will lead the way out and alleviate the fear experienced.

Being lost in the woods creates a constant anxiety that can easily turn into panic and the constant need to look for something familiar. There is another aspect to this experience - a loss of peripheral vision.

> You have been lost for two hours/
> You follow a bend in the trail
> Below you is a valley of beautiful flowers/
> Would you see them?

Probably not! While lost and experiencing considerable anxiety or panic, one seems to lose peripheral or side vision. In its place there develops what can be called narrow or tunnel vision. All energies become focused straight ahead in an attempt to determine where you are going and how to get out. Again, being lost creates - a constant anxiety that can easily turn into panic, looking for something familiar, and narrow or tunnel vision. The experience is still not complete.

> You and I are lost together in the woods/
> At the three hour point
> I say to you, "I am cold. I am scared. I am hungry."/
> Would you care?

Probably not! It is hard to be sensitive to what someone else is experiencing when you are encountering the same thing. People who become lost develop what can be called egocentric-like behavior. Experiencing a very small world causes a loss of sensitivity to people around them. While lost for an extended period, the incessant fear is for one's survival - "How will I make it through this?"

There are five components to being lost - a feeling of anxiety that can easily turn into panic, looking for something familiar, narrow/tunnel vision, egocentric-like behavior, and a fear for one's survival.

Exactly what it may be like to be mentally impaired!

a) Anxiety to Panic

A mentally impaired client is lost in a world that makes little sense. This experience causes a state of constant anxiety that can easily turn into panic. I am often asked, "How do you know the emotional state of the mentally impaired is so fragile?" Let me demonstrate:

Imagine:

> I approach you right now
> Place a blindfold over your eyes
> Plug your ears so you cannot hear/
> I take you to an unknown destination
> Telling you nothing of where you are going or why/
>
> I remove your blindfold and ear plugs
> You find yourself in an unfamiliar building/
> In a large crowded room with people you have never seen
> before/

I leave with instructions to those in the room not to let you
leave/
You can find nothing in the room to help you identify your
location/
The people who confront you speak a language you have never
heard before/
You find yourself unable to decipher any meaning from their
attempts to communicate with you/

People are constantly moving about
Some are touching your clothing
Placing you here, then there/
Even when you refuse to follow, they take you/
Your attempts to leave the building are always thwarted
At times their behavior seems quite bizarre and threatening/

It is getting dark
You believe your family should be missing you by now and
coming to get you/
Instead you are taken to a bedroom with two beds in it/
A person lies motionless in the bed by the door
No sound, no reaction to the activities around/
You are stripped of your clothing
And motioned to lie down on the empty bed/
The lights are turned out/

You cannot rest
You hear unfamiliar noises from outside the door/
Periodically in the darkness a figure walks into the room with a
flashlight
It is shone in your direction
Then the person leaves/

The sun rises/
Someone comes to you
Hands you a bowl with water and two pieces of cloth/
You do not understand what is asked/

4

The individual takes the cloth, places it in the water
And then moves the cloth to your face
You attempt to stop her but are unsuccessful/

You never know where you are/
Who the people are around you
Faces and things never remain constant/
The fear you experience never leaves you/
Each day the experience is the same/

What I have just described portrays admission to long term care for a mentally impaired older person. They feel constant and chronic anxiety that will easily turn into panic. When that panic state is reached, it creates for this individual significant distress, and becomes the major causative factor for aggressive outbursts.

It is easy to demonstrate how the anxiety of the mentally impaired can be peaked to a panic level. Imagine a mentally impaired resident of a long term care facility who has lived there for a year or longer. Even though she is confused and disoriented, she has gained considerable familiarity. She may not know where she is, but she can find her room. She does not know staff by name, but she can recognize some by face.

Take that same mentally impaired individual and place her on a bus for an outing. You will probably find that removing her from her familiar environment to one that is foreign may dramatically increase her confusion level and change her behavior. This demonstrates an important concept:

When the mentally impaired are moved
from the familiar to the unfamiliar,
anxiety will increase,
behavior may change and mental functioning may decrease.

This fragile emotional state of the mentally impaired and their hypersensitivity to change are significant aspects in our discussion on aggressive behavior. It is these concepts that become the basis for what will be described as the Aggressive Episode, the Chronic Aggressive Pattern and the Violent Episode.

5

[Note: At this time it is important to emphasize a point. The above example does not imply that the mentally impaired should not be involved in activities such as bus trips or any similar outing. As we will discuss in later chapters, there are four possible responses to such events, each requiring a different intervention strategy.]

b) Looking for Something Familiar

Return to the experience of being lost in the woods. Imagine:

> After two hours of being lost/
> You stumble onto a candy wrapper
> You know you dropped before you were lost/

> What would be your response to finding that candy wrapper?

The loss of recent memory and analytical ability are common symptoms experienced by the mentally impaired. Either of these can create for this person a state of chaos in any setting. The inability to remember where one is, and to analyze what is seen, can create significant distress. To be able to find something familiar will provide some security, a feeling of control, which in turn will alleviate much of the anxiety experienced. This need causes many mentally impaired clients to constantly look for something familiar - house, spouse, clothing, etc. in order to understand the environment around them.

This action describes well why many mentally impaired clients frequently misinterpret the cueing about them. Their need to understand where they are and what is happening requires them to find things and people that they can recognize. This will often lead to their misinterpreting objects and people around them - familiar objects belonging to others become theirs; strangers with familiar features become family members.

The distress created by the lack of familiarity within the environment, the constant need to find things that are familiar, the experience of being contradicted when those things are found (being told she is wrong about who a person is or who the object belongs to) - all of these become contributing factors to aggressive outbursts.

c) Narrow/Tunnel Vision

Similar to the experience of being lost, the mentally impaired also develop narrow or tunnel vision. Their loss of recent memory and analytical ability would exhaust them if they had to be attentive to everything around them. Their visual field needs to be focused in order to cope with their surroundings. This inability to handle _all_ stimuli creates a need to limit one's perceptual awareness. Without this narrowed or tunneled vision, the mentally impaired would feel bombarded, constantly overwhelmed by their environment. Instead they view their world as though looking through a tube or down a tunnel. This results in a loss of visual acuity from side-to-side, as well as above and below eye level.

To demonstrate this phenomenon, just sit two mentally impaired clients side-by-side. You will usually notice little if any interaction between the two of them. It appears as though they do not see each other. The inability to notice the other person is based on their need to focus on what is occurring straight ahead. The mentally impaired are drawn to every stimuli, noise and movement in front of them. They haven't the cognitive ability or energy level to concentrate on what is happening to the side of them as well. As will be demonstrated, this is an important concept in methods of approaching this person. If the approach is not adapted to this limitation, it will distress the individual and could lead to an aggressive response.

Diminished awareness of visual acuity above and below eye level can also be demonstrated. Many mentally impaired clients will look down as they walk, concentrating on where they are placing their feet. When they are not looking down, they will trip over the simplest things. Similarly, anything placed above eye level will often not be seen by the mentally impaired, and it becomes lost from view. This loss of peripheral vision will be significant when examining some of the _distressers_ that may lead to aggressive behavior.

d) Egocentric-Like Behavior

It is common to hear from the spouse of an Alzheimer's victim:

> "My wife and I have been married for 47 years. In that entire period whenever I was feeling physically unwell, she would help me every chance she got. Whenever I was hurting emotionally, she would hold me. Since she has become impaired, it doesn't matter how sick I am, she never helps. It doesn't matter how much I hurt, she never holds me."

It would be impossible to relate to the needs and feelings of others when you are in a state of chaos yourself. How could you be sensitive towards someone else when you are unable to understand or control what is happening around you? The mentally impaired develop an egocentric-like behavior, a very small world, overwhelmed by their own feelings. This experience along with their loss of analytical ability explains why the mentally impaired become very self-centered in any stressful situation.

e) Survival

For this person there can only exist one basic need - survival. The fear, the confusion, the lack of familiarity all contribute to an overwhelming sensitivity to circumstances around them. It is this need that will initiate their dramatic response when the feeling of being out of control is intensified.

We have now established the basic foundation for aggressive behavior of the mentally impaired. The overall experience creates for them a state where aggression, wandering or withdrawal are common coping strategies in any stressful situation. By understanding these concepts we can appreciate the intervention strategies needed to provide the controls required.

UNDERSTANDING THEIR VULNERABILITY

Return again to the experience of being lost in the woods. I want you to imagine the following:

As soon as you become lost
I appear/
You have never seen me before/
You do not know why I am there/

I follow you for the entire four hours that you are lost
I am always forty steps behind you/
You walk forward, I move with you
You come towards me, I go the other way
You try and talk to me, I do not answer/

How are you now?

Encountering an unknown stimuli at a time when you are experiencing a great deal of anxiety, will elevate that anxiety to its highest degree. The confusion created by what is occurring can result in one of three responses:

You could become highly agitated,
prepared to fight the person who appears as a threat to you
or
You could run away blindly trying to get away from this person
or
You could sit down and cry, becoming totally paralyzed by the threat

When emotions peak to a panic state, problem solving, analytical thought, coping ability, behavior, etc. are all impacted. You will find yourself in a crisis state where effective coping ability has been negated. This leaves you with only one of three responses:

fight - *attempt to defend yourself from the stresser.*
flight - *attempt to remove yourself from the stresser.*
withdraw - *surrender to the stresser.*

9

Change the scenario.

> You are mentally impaired/
> Very confused and disoriented/
> You are sitting in a chair in your room
> It is 9:15 in the morning/
>
> A person you do not know enters your room/
> She steps behind you to straighten your bed
> While there, she asks, "Do you have to go to the bathroom?"/
> You do not know who she is talking to
> Or understand what she is saying
> You do not answer/
>
> Suddenly that person steps in front of you/
> Takes you by the arm
> Lifts you from the chair/
> You do not know who she is/
> You do not know where she is taking you/
>
> How would you respond?

There is nothing different from this encounter than the one described previously while lost in the woods. You have three possible responses:

> fight her - *aggressive response*
> try to get away from her - *wandering response*
> become paralyzed, allowing her to do what she wants -
>   *withdrawal response*

This scenario demonstrates many of the *distresser*s that can illicit either of these responses.

- you did not know who the person was (you lacked rapport or trust).
- she was talking to you from behind.
- the question was not directed to you.

- you were unable to understand who she was talking to and what she was saying.
- the staff member's actions occurred too fast and without warning.
- you did not have enough time to analyze what she was doing and why.

This emphasizes three very important concepts about the mentally impaired -

1) When a stimuli is not intense enough it will be misinterpreted (made to fit their reality) or missed (not seen or heard).

2) The mentally impaired require time to process information.

3) To be successful with this clientele, rapport or trust must be established with every contact.

This scenario demonstrates that with many simple interactions:

the thought process of the mentally impaired
may not have enough time to catch up
with the actions of the caregiver.

The actions of the staff member only confused you further - you did not know who she was or where she was taking you. When your confusion was increased, it intensified your feeling of being out of control. That pushed your anxiety level to a panic state and caused you to become aggressive, wander or withdraw. We have just established the premise for the *Aggressive Pattern* of the mentally impaired.

Anything that confuses the mentally impaired further
(called a *circumstantial episode*)
Increases their feeling of being out of control
Pushes their anxiety level to a panic state
Causes them to become aggressive, wander or withdraw

This concept will be expanded in detail throughout the following chapters. As we will discover, it is this pattern that becomes the most common cause for the majority of aggressive outbursts of the mentally impaired.

Comparing the scenario of being lost in the woods with the experience of being mental impaired is helpful. It provides something the caregiver can relate to that will allow clearer understanding of this person's experience. The better we can understand that experience, the better we can adjust our supports and interventions accordingly.

Although this comparison is effective, it has its limitations. Being lost in the woods and the subsequent effects are sequential and logical. The emotions elicited, as well as the impact on problem solving and thinking ability, maintain some rationality. The experience of being mentally impaired probably does not have that benefit. It possesses no logic or rationality. Losing analytical ability and recent memory retention can only create a state of chaos. Our challenge as caregivers is to find something that will help us to understand this person's world. The better it can be understood, the more we are able to assist this person to cope with an unbearable situation.

It is important now to examine the disease, its symptomology, the levels of care and the person's vulnerability to external factors.

THE TERM MENTAL IMPAIRMENT

In this text you will find the term Alzheimer's disease used sparingly. In its place will be the term mental impairment. Mental impairment implies that there is more than just one disease involved and that all parts of the brain can be affected.

Let us address the former issue. Alzheimer's disease is only one of many diseases with similar symptomology and progression. The following diseases all have a similar clinical picture as Alzheimer's, but have different causative factors or biological dynamics.

> Pick's Disease
> Frontal Lobe Degeneration, Non-Alzheimer's Type
> Progressive Subcortical Gliosis
> ALS - Dementia Syndrome

Adult Onset Intranuclear Hyaline Inclusion Disease
Hereditary Dysphasic Dementia
Posterior Cerebral Atrophy
Creutzfieldt-Jacob Disease
Lewy Body Dementia
Joseph's Disease

And there are still more! The majority of these diseases can only be definitively diagnosed on autopsy. The symptoms they generate, how they progress, the vulnerability they create and their general patterns (the clinical picture) have many similar qualities. Although Alzheimer's disease is the most dominant, the term mental impairment becomes all inclusive to demonstrate that we are dealing with a specific state or experience, not a specific disease process.

The second reason for employing the term mental impairment is to demonstrate the full range of the destructive process that can occur within the brain. The frequently employed phrase *cognitive dysfunctioning* seems too limiting. It implies that there is only a loss in thinking ability. In actual fact, all mental functioning can be impaired, including physical abilities. Mental impairment seems more appropriate in defining the actual extent of the damage that occurs.

To understand the biological changes that occurs with all of the diseases related to mental impairment would be too consuming. The focus of this text is not on the disease process, but on its effects. Therefore, we will only focus on Alzheimer's disease in our discussion of the destructive process that occurs.

THE CLINICAL PICTURE

Alzheimer's disease demonstrates a specific quality -

progressive deterioration of mental functioning until death.

The loss of mental ability caused by the disease process appears as follows:

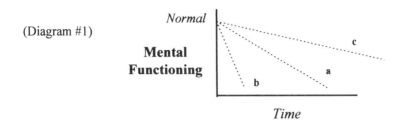

(Diagram #1)

Mental Functioning — *Normal*

Time

The three dotted lines on the graph demonstrates clinical examples of the deterioration that can occur. Showing more than one dotted line illustrates the individualization that is experienced. The rate of destruction within the brain and the speed of deterioration can vary from individual to individual.

A common slang term used by lay people when referring to this disease is "old people's disease." Unfortunately that belief is inaccurate. This disease can strike anyone over the age of forty. Some cases have even involved individuals in their twenties. Under the age of sixty-five, the disease is commonly referred to as Pre-senile Alzheimer's. The progression of the disease for the younger person is often very rapid, with an average life expectancy after onset of two years. The line marked as 'b' on the graph represents the speed at which the deterioration can occur with this age group. The person under sixty-five generally shows dramatic change over a short period of time.

For those over sixty-five years of age the disease is referred to as Senile Dementia of the Alzheimer's Type. The average life expectancy for the older person after onset is eight years. Some can live over twenty years with the disease (line 'c' on the graph). The slower the disease progress, the more gradual the changes that occur.

It is important to emphasize that the progression of the disease, as with everything else with this disease, is highly individualized. The disease possesses little predictability in how quickly it will progress, what symptoms will be encountered, how long it will last, etc. The numerical statistics stated are based on the average. In actual fact, the disease can last only a few short years for some, to a few decades for others, regardless of age.

THE BIOLOGICAL CHANGES

This disease represents brain damage to its ultimate extent! In fact the brain of an Alzheimer's victim may shrink up to 40% in weight and in size by the time of death.

When most think of damage to the brain at an older age, they often associate it with a dysfunction in the circulatory system. With Alzheimer's that is not so much the case. Instead brain cells of an Alzheimer's victim are destroyed. The disease causes certain neurons to deteriorate, taking on a peculiar shape and eventually losing their ability to function.

Microscopic views of damaged neurons show nerve cells that "appear to be tied into knots." These configurations are called neurofibril tangles. At some point these cells are completely destroyed, causing black patches of dead tissue throughout certain regions of the brain called senile plaques.

These changes can cause varying degrees of destruction and can be located <u>anywhere</u> in the brain. The predominant areas seem to be the temporal and frontal lobes, and the heart of the brain called the hippocampus. This presents an important consequence relevant to caring for an Alzheimer's victim.

The location and degree of damage is individualized.

This dictates that no two Alzheimer's victims are identical in the degree and location of destruction within the brain. Therefore there are no two Alzheimer's victims who will experience the same intensity and pattern of symptoms. As a result, programming needs are also individualized. What will work for one Alzheimer's victim, may not work for another.

One of the most important concepts that can be gained from understanding this disease is:

What is lost is lost, you cannot put it back.
There is no way to stop this disease, cure it or at this time to slow it down.

15

UNDERSTANDING THE DAMAGE PROCESS

This disease is highly unique. Not only may large areas within the brain be destroyed, but small groupings of cells may also be involved. These small groupings of cells can be called Pin Point Areas of Destruction.

When major areas of the brain are damaged, the needs and approach are obvious. For example, if 90% of the area that controls the ability to recognize names and faces is destroyed, you do not need an assessment tool to uncover it. Your initial contact with this individual will quickly identify his limitation. When a specific area of the brain is severely damaged, it is obvious that the challenge is to determine what functioning ability still remains.

Yet it is still not that simple. What about the situation where 90% of an area is still functioning and only 10% is damaged? The loss of that ability is not so obvious. If the assessment tools are not in place to uncover the 10% that is lost, then it creates significant distress that will result in an aggressive response. The following examples will demonstrate the complexity that can occur.

An Alzheimer's victim may be able to dress himself when his shirt, pants, socks and shoes are placed in front of him. When a pullover sweater is placed in front of him, he only stares at it. Caregivers who do not understand the dynamics of this disease, sometimes misinterpret such behavior as resistive or attention seeking. They believe that if he is able to dress himself with other articles of clothing, he should be able to put this one on as well. They interpret his behavior as intentional, a premeditated act "to be difficult" and may pressure him to put the sweater on himself. The result is obvious - he will become aggressive.

If the cells within the brain that retain the imagery or picture of what a sweater looks like are destroyed, then the picture is lost. To this person a sweater is a foreign object. He responds to it as though he has never seen it before. He experiences what can be called agnosia, the loss of association to a specific object.

It can become even more complex. He may know what a pullover sweater looks like, but does not know how to put it on. He cannot identify the top, the bottom, the left or the right. He has lost the mechanics of how to manipulate the sweater.

It even becomes more complex. You pull out a chair, pat the seat and say, "Please sit in the chair." He sits down. A half hour later he walks into the room and you simply say, "Please sit in the chair." He does not respond. The reason for his lack of response may be that he does not know the meaning of the word "chair." When he sees one, he knows what to do with it. What it is called he cannot remember. He has lost the ability to associate a word to a specific object.

In one facility when staff stood a lady in front of the toilet and stated, "Please sit down on the toilet." She would not sit down. When they turned her around to let her look at the toilet, she would then sit on it.

These subtle losses in functioning ability must be uncovered. Without defining them, we can inadvertently pressure an individual to function at a level that is beyond her ability. This pressuring will in turn result in an aggressive response. It is easy to demonstrate the associated frustrations that can occur.

> Would you pick up your sforten full of gotterfek
> And place it by your swaskart.

You haven't the slightest idea what I am referring to. But if you lost the ability to recognize certain objects by name, saying "glass" would have no more meaning than referring to it as your "sforten," or the word "orange juice" communicate anymore to you than a "gotterfek" and "plate" tell you anything more than "swaskart."

When it is not known what you can comprehend, then it is easy to repeatedly pressure you to perform what appears as a simple task. In order to prevent Alzheimer's aggression, the strengths and limitations of the individual must be defined.

THE CARE PROCESS

What has been outlined about the biological changes to this point establishes a significant aspect of how this disease and the symptoms must be viewed.

If you have a symptom of an Alzheimer's victim that can be stopped
with something other than medication
then it is not Alzheimer's that is causing it.

If *enough* dosage of a drug is administered, it can mask any behavior, usually to the detriment of the client.

On the contrary, if it were so easy to stop the symptoms, why would that person need to be admitted to a long term care facility. Any symptom related to the biological changes occurring within the brain cannot be stopped. They can only be made tolerable for those who must live or work with this individual and for the client herself to decrease her distress. This becomes the intervention focus required to prevent Alzheimer's aggression.

Knowing that this is brain damage, defines well the approach involved in caring for this clientele. It is called *common sense*. Unfortunately, it is impossible to sell common sense as a viable intervention focus and still have credibility in the health care milieu. It seems that health care has deemed only "therapies" to be effective. So I have called this philosophy of care *Supportive Therapy*.

This concept is based on the biological changes that occur. Given that this is brain damage, what is lost is lost and it cannot be replaced, there are only two approaches that can be taken.

1) *Identify for this person his strengths, what he is still able to do and maintain them.*
2) *Identify his limitations, what he can no longer do and compensate for them.*

This must be done for this person for the rest of his life, knowing that his situation will only worsen with time (Diagram #1).

People who do not understand this clientele believe there is little that can be done for them. There may be little that can be done about the disease, but there is a great deal that can be done to help the person cope with what is occurring.

THE LEVELS OF FUNCTIONING

Alzheimer's disease is progressive in nature. In order to understand the specific target group that is most vulnerable for aggressive behavior, it is important to summarize the levels of functioning detailed in the text The Tactics of Supportive Therapy (Book One).

Level One - Mild
- Physically well.
- Symptoms are mild, and can be easily compensated for.
- Still mentally high functioning.
- Usually living at home.
- Aware of something being wrong or that she/he has the disease.
- Major challenge involves the mood swings created by the grieving process.

Level Two - Moderate
- Highly confused and disoriented.
- Does not view self as sick.
- Usually physically well and ambulatory.
- Demonstrates a variety of symptoms, including loss of analytical ability.
- Unable to care for self.
- Requires constant supervision.
- Usually living in a long term care facility.
- Major challenges are behavioral - wandering and aggression.
- Experiences Reality Conflict, where two worlds seem to be going on at the same time, yours and theirs, both are in conflict.

Level Three - Severe
- Very incapacitated, both physically and mentally.
- Needs total care (washed, fed, dressed, etc.).
- Incontinent.
- Non-ambulatory.
- Limited communicative ability.
- Limited awareness of surroundings.

Rather than distinct levels, the progression must be viewed more as a continuum. As the disease worsens, some mentally impaired will have characteristics of Level One. At some point they will possess qualities of both Level One and Two. As it worsens further, they will demonstrate the characteristics of Level Two. Again as the disease progresses, they will assimilate some of the qualities of both Levels Two and Three, and then finally move into Level Three. There is no way to predict how long a person will remain in each level. As everything else with this disease, it is highly individualized.

The emphasis in this text is on Level Two. It is this person who is the most challenging. Level One still has some understanding of his environment and retains some rational ability to enhance his coping. Level Three is the least sensitive to environmental stimuli and usually that stimuli can be easily removed.

Level two on the other hand is highly sensitive. The loss of analytical ability and recent memory retention makes this individual the most vulnerable to the circumstances encountered. This person's reaction when distressed is to become aggressive, wander or withdraw. Once programming for Level Two has been defined, it can be adapted to fit the needs of those in Level One and Three.

THE SYMPTOMS

There are many symptoms associated with mental impairment. Many of these symptoms are outlined in detail in the text The Tactics of Supportive Therapy. Below is a brief list and description of those symptoms that play a significant part in understanding the aggressive outbursts of the mentally impaired.

Symptom	Description
Judgment	Loss of the analytical ability to define extremes - good/bad, right/wrong, too much/too little.
Orientation - place	Interprets the cues based on the person's perception of the situation.
- person	Some can remember names and faces, some only faces and some neither.
- time	Cannot remember a stationary point from which to measure the passage of time, therefore may only be able to recall events.
- thing	Loss of ability to identify objects or associate specific words to objects.
Memory - Recent & Past	Memory is selective, only remember events that have attached to them significant emotions either positive or negative.
Affect - Flat	Loss of spontaneous emotional expression causing masked a facial expression, rarely laughs or cries.
- Volatile	Explosive, sitting quietly, with no warning will become violent, for no reason will stop
Persistent Stimuli - speech - motor - tactile - pain	Repetitive behaviors due to damaged cells within specific locations of the brain.

Loss of Cognition	Loss of analytical ability to maintain sequential though, impairing problem solving.
Progressive Apraxia	Loss of purposeful muscle movement.
Progressive Aphasia	Word substitution to loss of vocabulary, gradually losing ability to communicate.
Illusion Behavior	Often incorrectly defined as hallucinatory behavior. Caused when the stimuli is not intense enough, it is misinterpreted and then made to fit this person's reality.
Rummaging & Hoarding	Caused by the lack of environmental differentiation or past behavior.
Delusions	Incorrect beliefs that are not based on reality, but with the mentally impaired, they are based on their reality and stimuli interpretation.
Mimicking	If the stimuli is too intense, some mentally impaired cannot help but respond. Some will mimic everything and anything - sitting, aggressive behavior, calling out, wandering, etc.

The symptoms encountered with Alzheimer's disease are varied and complex. They will mimic almost any other disease that affects the central nervous system. The majority of other non-dementia diseases are more localized, impacting on only limited areas of the brain. Hence the symptoms encountered are often limited and more predictable. The diseases that cause mental impairment are more generalized. They can affect almost every part of the brain. Therefore almost any symptom can be experienced. The programming strategies must be broad and all encompassing. This emphasizes the need for the caregiver to be flexible in being able to adapt to the individual client and that person's uniqueness.

There are two symptoms that must be detailed to allow further discussion of Alzheimer's aggression and methods of approaching this individual. They are volatile affect and progressive apraxia.

VOLATILE AFFECT

This is the <u>biological cause</u> of violent behavior. It is seen in a mentally impaired client who is sitting quietly and for no apparent reason becomes violent. This violent behavior will sometimes last twenty seconds and other times up to twenty minutes or longer before it stops.

The cause of this phenomenon is unique to the destructive process of the disease. As mentioned earlier, the cells within the brain may be damaged before they are destroyed. During this time, they become distorted and may change their functioning ability. This change may create a type of hyperactivity, where the affected cells can "fire off" an electrical impulse easily and stimulate that area of the brain.

These dynamics can be compared to epilepsy. It is not suggested that epilepsy and Alzheimer's are the same, but the biological changes occurring with epilepsy may demonstrate a similar outcome as Alzheimer's. In epilepsy there is an alteration to specific brain tissue. These "changed" cells have the ability to "fire off" on their own, stimulating the brain and causing a grand mal seizure. Once the grand mal seizure has begun, there is nothing that can be done to stop it. At that time, the person must be made safe, and the seizure allowed to run its course until it is over.

The symptom of volatile affect may be similar. Certain cells in the area of the brain that control emotional expression may have been damaged, but not yet destroyed. They have the ability to "fire off" on their own, stimulating that area of the brain. This results in the person virtually going into what can be considered an "emotional seizure."

Unfortunately, all that can be done when this occurs is to empty the room, back off, keep that person and others safe and let it run its course. An individual with this symptom is usually sedated because of the unpredictability of the violent outbursts. Family are unable to care for this person at home, and neither can staff of most long term care facilities effectively deal with this individual. This person is best cared for in a specialized psychiatric facility or unit. The primary focus taken by this setting is to find a medication regime that is effective without creating further complications.

The symptom of volatile affect is *not common* with the Alzheimer's victim. That is not to say that a mentally impaired client cannot be

pushed to violence. The difference between volatile affect and circumstantial episodes that will lead to violent behavior are the absence of what will be explained as "The Behavioral Pattern." Volatile affect does not seem to have a pattern. It seems to appear regardless of the time of day or what is occurring around or to the person. Circumstantial episodes that lead to a violent response always demonstrate a behavioral pattern, indicating that something has happened to "trigger" the outburst to occur.

PROGRESSIVE APRAXIA

This symptom involves the loss of coordinated muscle movement. The mentally impaired affected by this symptom still know how to cognitively perform a task, but can no longer coordinate muscle movement in order to complete it. The progression of this symptom can be observed. Initially the person will be able to feed herself with a fork and a knife. As time passes, she will only be able to use a fork, then only a spoon, then her fingers, then she will stop feeding herself completely. She has moved from fine motor movement ability to only gross motor movement.

Progressive apraxia is the common reason the mentally impaired will be unable to walk. It is unusual for a mentally impaired person to be walking one day and no longer able to walk the next (except for a secondary problem such as a fractured hip). Instead the loss of muscle coordination results in losing the ability to maintain balance necessary for walking.

Again, the deterioration of ability can be viewed. The person will walk without difficulty. As the disease progresses, she will begin falling periodically. Over time, her falling will increase to where she is unable to walk only a few steps without assistance. At this point she has either injured herself (i.e. with a fractured hip) and is unable to walk or has been restricted to a chair for her own safety.

There are many examples that demonstrate this loss of muscle control.

- Some mentally impaired will need to "glide down the hall" in order to reach their destination. They will use the wall to support them as they walk. This demonstrates the importance of an unobstructed hallway and large hand rails along the wall for the person to grasp.

- Many mentally impaired clients even fight balance while sitting in a chair. This is why they will usually not sit in chairs without arm rests for extended periods of time. As soon as they try to relax, they will lose their balance and lean to the side. When there are no arm rests, the person will feel as though she is falling out of the chair, jerk herself back up to a sitting position and then get out of the chair. Arm rests, on the other hand, will support her as she leans, making her feel more secure and allowing her to sit for longer periods.

- Many mentally impaired clients will employ a rocking motion when getting out of a chair. They can no longer coordinate the needed muscle groupings to lift themselves out of the chair. The rocking motion gives them enough momentum to push themselves out. This explains why they can become distressed in low chairs, recliners or chairs where the seat is too soft. These chairs have a restraining effect, making it difficult for them to stand. Chairs with higher than normal seats allow them to stand with the least effort. Likewise, chairs with arm rests allows the person to push up to the standing position.

- Progressive apraxia is also one of the reasons many mentally impaired clients cannot turn sharply while walking, or are reluctant to move around obstacles. When coordination is lost, the ability to maintain one's center of gravity is also impaired. To turn or side step changes their center of gravity. Once it is altered, they have difficulty regaining it, causing them to lose their balance and fall. This explains one of the reasons why they are more apt to move obstacles out of their way (wheelchairs, chairs, etc.) or bowl people over who stand in front of them, rather than walk around them. In fact in one long term care facility, a mentally impaired resident was found in a laundry hamper - back end in the hamper, feet and arms pointing to the sky. The laundry room was very small. When he entered, he had no where to go. When he turned around he had nothing to hold onto, lost his balance and fell back into the hamper. It was quite a sight.

Progressive apraxia must be taken into consideration when considering environmental design, as well as the strategies employed when approaching the mentally impaired. Each of these will be discussed in detail in the upcoming chapters.

We have discussed to this point the biological process of Alzheimer's disease and examined the experience of being mentally impaired. Neither of these explains the more sudden changes in behavior and ability. Some mentally impaired clients are able to function at a certain level one day and differently the next. In fact some are able to complete certain tasks at one time of the day and not the next. This now leads us to outlining the vulnerability to *Secondary Factors* that this disease process creates.

THE SECONDARY FACTORS

There are two causes for every behavior of the mentally impaired
- biological and circumstantial.

The circumstantial episodes are created by what can be called Secondary Factors. Anything that fits the following criteria constitutes a Secondary Factor :

⇒ impairs the person's mental abilities further.
⇒ creates abrupt changes in behavior or functioning ability.

⇒ is not directly related to the disease process causing mental impairment.

⇒ is treatable or reversible.

Diagram #2 demonstrates the potential changes in functioning that can occur when Secondary Factors are encountered. The deterioration in functioning ability caused by the disease process is represented by the dotted line (marked as 'a'). The sudden drop in functioning level (solid line, marked as 'b') represents the effect of a Secondary Factor.

(Diagram #2)

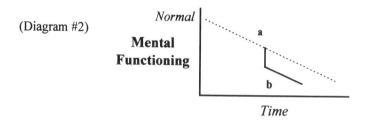

Mental Functioning

Normal

a

b

Time

The Secondary Factors that can create these effects are drugs, disease, approach and environment. Any of these have the ability to change this person's behavior and functioning ability if not corrected.

DRUGS

The sensitivity of older people to medication has been a long standing concern. The mentally impaired elderly are significantly more sensitive to medication than the older population in general. This makes medication use with the mentally impaired a major consideration.

The negative impact of certain medications on the elderly can be dramatic. We know little about the effects of one drug on an older person let alone a combination of possibly five, eight or ten different medications taken in a twenty-four hour period.

This sensitivity is compounded even further with the mentally impaired elderly. In fact, their reaction to any one drug may be as great as four times what is experienced by the older population in general.

With any mentally impaired client, functioning on all counts can deteriorate dramatically given the wrong medication at the wrong time.

Whenever a mentally impaired client's behavior changes or functioning level deteriorates (whether physically, mentally or emotionally) the first questions that must be asked are:

> What change has been made to the dose or times of medications given?
> What new drug has been ordered?

If a recent change in medication has occurred, then that is the first area to be investigated as its possible cause. Examples of medication sensitivity will be detailed with the case study presented in the next chapter.

DISEASE

> What is the effect on the mental state of a mentally impaired client who experiences a bout of the flu - diarrhea or upper respiratory tract infection?

In many cases her mental functioning will decrease, her confusion and disorientation will increase (a drop in functioning as noted in line 'b', diagram #2). You know yourself when you experience an upper respiratory tract infection you have difficulty breathing, you are lethargic, you cannot think clearly or quickly. Your own functioning ability decreases. With the mentally impaired, any subtle change in functioning ability will show dramatic symptomology. Cure that acute infection and the person's functioning will return to her original state of the disease (line 'a', diagram #2).

Any physical disease process can have similar results. A mentally impaired individual with controlled congestive heart failure experiences an acute bout of that condition - short of breath, diaphoretic (severe sweating), cyanotic (bluish coloration of the skin), etc. During that time and even for some time after he is re-stabilized, there will be an obvious decline in his cognitive ability. The acute episode affects the blood-oxygen flow to the brain, thereby decreasing the brain's performance, and potentially increasing the level of confusion experienced. Stabilizing the congestive heart failure will return him to his original functioning state (line 'a', diagram #2).

The organic changes experienced by the brain of a person with Alzheimer's Disease can create considerable sensitivity to alterations in any body process. The brain's effectiveness to perform can be hampered by changes to any of the major organs of the body - liver, heart, lungs, circulatory system, kidneys, etc.

Even the slightest physical change can show dramatic variation in ability. When a mentally impaired person does not sleep one night, his functioning ability during the next day will have deteriorated and his behavior changed. Tasks he could easily perform the day before, he will be unable to do today.

Constipation, hemorrhoids, any physical discomfort or pain will have the same results. If the care environment in which this person lives does not accurately assess these changes in ability and behavior, then those performing the care will not possess the flexibility to adapt this person's routine and tasks to accommodate what has happened. This will result in the client being pressured to perform at a level beyond his ability, causing an aggressive outburst.

APPROACH

> You are mentally impaired
> Sitting in your chair/
> At 0845 hours I enter your room
> To take you to the bathroom/
> Standing over you I ask, "Do you have to go to the washroom?"/
> Without any further direction
> I take you by the elbow to assist you to stand
> You resist, becoming aggressive and defensive/

If the agitation created by this event ended when the caregiver left the room, there would be little problem. That is not always the case. Instead it is more common that the heightened level of fear and anxiety will remain. With some clients it can last for hours, with others the rest of the day.

In fact, this heightened fear and anxiety could spill over to other staff, situations and other shifts. That one event could affect the success of any staff. During that day, even those who normally have little difficulty taking you to the washroom, may now find you difficult to handle.

Once the anxiety level of the mentally impaired client is increased, it may take some time for a sense of security to return. During this heightened anxiety state, there exists a strong suspicious tendency when interpreting the actions of others. Normal tasks and performance levels will be dramatically affected during this period (line 'b', diagram #2).

This effect can be demonstrated further.

If I approached you at 1130 hours in the manner described above, causing you to become agitated, what would be your response when I place your lunch in front of you at 1200 hours?

I would hope that I had another clean uniform - I may be wearing your lunch.

You know well the effects of a staff member who employs an inappropriate approach when caring for the mentally impaired. If you can arrive on duty at seven in the morning and know exactly who was working the previous night shift by the number of mentally impaired residents who are agitated and/or wandering, then you have identified the effect. The change in a resident's behavior is often due to the elevated anxiety created by the approach and environment encountered. Once one's anxiety level is increased, mental functioning deteriorates. The resident is now unable to perform tasks he could easily perform under more supportive circumstances.

In fact one of the assessment tools used to investigate serious aggressive or violent episodes within a long term care facility, is to examine who was caring for this individual the previous sixteen hours. We will identify that not all health care professionals are capable of caring for this type of individual effectively. Those who lack understanding of the disease, who do not possess the needed insights to pick up behavioral cueing, who are not prepared to be flexible in their care routine, etc. can be highly detrimental to the mentally impaired. The pressuring they create over an eight hour period may be enough to illicit a highly intense response by specific mentally impaired clients. This will be demonstrated in detail in the upcoming chapters.

ENVIRONMENT

If you work in a long term care setting, is there a difference on your unit Sunday morning at 1000 hours versus Monday morning at 1000 hours?

In many long term care facilities, Sunday mornings can be quite quiet. Monday mornings, on the other hand, seem to be when everyone is doing almost anything, all at the same time. During that period the unit can be quite hectic.

You know what I am talking about on those days when you leave the unit at the end of your shift saying to yourself "Thank God I am out of there. I was going crazy with what was going on." If we become stressed by the noise and commotion, then the mentally impaired become highly distressed.

The floor plan below (diagram #3) is of a long term care unit housing forty-four mentally impaired residents.

(Diagram #3)

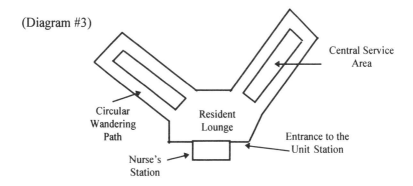

Central Service Area

Circular Wandering Path

Resident Lounge

Entrance to the Unit Station

Nurse's Station

The unit contained a large resident lounge in front of the nurse's station where the majority of the residents sat during the day. The main entrance to the unit was located at one end of the lounge. The two wings each housed approximately twenty-two residents. Each wing had a circular wandering path that went through the lounge.

Residents normally sat around the walls and in the center of the lounge. All traffic traveled through the lounge - laundry carts, wanderers, medication cart, maintenance staff, housekeeping staff, nursing staff, recreation staff, visitors, volunteers, and so on. During the height of the activity (from 0830 to 1200 hours on the day shift) the comings and goings that occurred in and around that lounge were intense. Likewise the aggressive outbursts during that time and for hours later were frequent.

Staff were aware of some of the commotion, but not its full intensity. They did not sit in the lounge for extended periods of time to allow themselves to become fully conscious of the amount of chaos encountered. The residents on that unit, on the other hand, were bombarded with that stimuli day in and day out.

The sensitivity of the mentally impaired to the environment is very significant. In fact it is possible to change the functioning ability and behavior of a mentally impaired older client within minutes. Simply conduct a fire drill. During a fire drill everyone is scurrying around, closing doors, herding people about, alarms are clanging. A short time later, everything is over. For the staff it may be over, but for some mentally impaired it has just begun. The chaos created by the activity and noise of a fire drill confuses some mentally impaired. They cannot understand the increased activity and commotion. This heightened confusion elevates their feeling of being out of control. That pushes their anxiety to a panic level and the person will become aggressive, wander or withdraw.

There are scores of examples of the impact of the environment. One unit housed thirty mentally impaired residents. During the night shift eleven of them were up, awake and agitated at 0200 hours. Their agitated state did not settle until 1400 hours that day. A half hour later, a group of five professionals toured the unit. They spent only fifteen minutes on the unit, walking about, talking to some of the residents and then they left. The behavior and change in functioning that existed before 1400 hours re-occurred shortly after their exodus. The added unknown stimuli was enough to re-ignite the distress of the mentally impaired who had not slept the night before.

We will discuss in detail some of the environmental strategies that can be employed to control the stimuli experienced by the mentally impaired. If they are not controlled, staff are left to deal with the consequences - aggressive outbursts.

The Secondary Factors that create the circumstantial episodes will be discussed in detail in the upcoming chapters. They are the premise for what will be defined as the Aggressive Episode, the Chronic Aggressive Pattern and the Violent Episode.

The concept of *Supportive Therapy* has demonstrated two care components in its assessment, programming and intervention strategies. One involves dealing with the biological changes that occur as result of the disease process. The care focus is supportive - identifying the strengths and maintaining them, identifying the limitations and compensating for them. The other component defines assessment tools, programming and intervention strategies that will eliminate the Secondary Factors that cause a circumstantial episode. The care focus is intervention.

SUMMARY

That last paragraph demonstrates well the challenges in working with this clientele. Once the limitations are defined, they must be supported for the rest of that person's life. That means the caregiver will be doing the same things over and over again with no improvement in this person's ability in that area. Likewise, his strengths or what he is still able to do will soon be lost and become limitations, requiring further care and support.

Given this fact, the successful care process requires ongoing assessment - functional tools that define this individual's abilities and recognizes when they become limitations. The emphasis must also be on the caregiver's perspective. The effective caregiver must possess a high energy level to maintain this person's independence regardless of the losses encountered; an enthusiasm to maintain the needed supports regardless of their repetitiveness; and a compassion to be sensitive to this person's vulnerability. There is no other way to assist this person through the losses encountered.

When the supports and intervention strategies are not adequately provided, it will lead to major aggressive response. The following chapter outlines a case example of how that can so easily occur.

Chapter Two

CASE EXAMPLE

Considerable time has been spent to this point defining the symptomology and vulnerability of the mentally impaired. The following case best demonstrates the dynamics creating circumstantial episodes, and defines the aggressive pattern presented by the mentally impaired elderly.

On hearing the details of this case, some are too quick to criticize those who cared for this individual and the long term care facility where he lived. In actual fact, that criticism is unjust. This case is not unique. It depicts many of the issues that face long term care today. The staff of this facility were doing the best they could with what they knew, and what they had available to them. No one can fault them for that.

Some of the specifics about this case have been altered slightly to ensure the anonymity of the organization in question. It is important to emphasize that this facility was quick to correct the identified problems, and to develop the necessary program strategies and staff supports to prevent similar experiences from occurring again.

Base line data about the unit in question:

- This was a 28 bed unit of a large facility.
- The unit was located on the third floor.
- There were no alarm or security devices on any of the doors exiting off the unit.
- The only alarms were located on the doors to the outside, located at the bottom of the stairs.
- This unit was constructed to accommodate cognitively well, physically disabled clients.

- The resident population was mixed with both mentally impaired and cognitively well, physically disabled residents.
- Staff were well trained and very skilled in dealing with the cognitively well, physically disabled residents.
- The care routines were developed years previously to accommodate the physically disabled and were not adapted as the clientele changed.

For this case, some of the functional assessment tools described later in the text were utilized. The assessment of the client in question was conducted over a two day period while consulting with the organization. The actual interview with the mentally impaired resident was the last part of the assessment. It occurred late during the second day. The period prior was invested in observing his behavior, attempting to establish rapport and gaining the significant preliminary data from staff and the chart (family were not available).

The floor plan of the unit appeared as follows:

(Diagram #4)

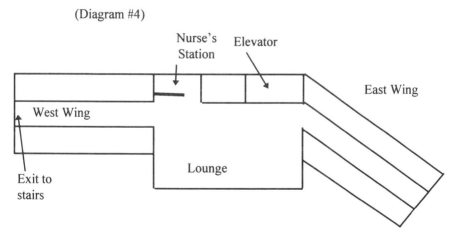

The assessment took place in April. Some base line data about the resident in question:

- male
- age 75 years old
- appeared much older
- quite frail physically
- experienced hypertension (elevated blood pressure)
- weighed 130 pounds
- tall in stature
- slim physique
- described as very confused and disoriented
- a wanderer who would periodically leave the building

One of the first assessment questions asked was - *Identify a time in the recent past when this person looked, acted or functioned differently than what would be seen today.* The staff identified that time as November of the previous year (six months earlier).

Prior to November, the resident walked with a full and normal gait, full extended stride, maintaining balance and arms swinging to his side. Up to November, when his wandering became disruptive, he could be directed to wipe off tables located in the lounge. Some staff stated that they were reluctant to encourage that behavior, because once he began, he would then wipe every table he could see, knocking off whatever was on top.

This gentleman had a very short attention span. He was able to concentrate on tasks for no more than four or five minutes. He was a mimicker, highly sensitive to stimuli and easily drawn to any noise, activity or movement on the unit (called *attractors*). He would stay with that *attractor* briefly, lose his concentration and then move on. He occasionally left the unit (eloped) when he wandered to the end of the hallway.

THE WANDERING PATTERN

It is important to differentiate the two types of elopement behavior (attempting to leave the building) that can occur with the mentally impaired. There is the *aggressive* eloper and the *incidental* eloper.

The *aggressive* eloper is not common. This individual is highly exhausting for any caregiver. This mentally impaired client will go through the exit door constantly. As soon as the caregiver returns this person to her chair, she is back to the door again. Even a secured unit will have difficulty managing this person's behavior. She is constantly by the door. Whenever the door is opened, she will bowl past whoever is entering or leaving the unit. If this person succeeds in leaving the building, she is traveling full speed down the street and is very difficult to return to the building.

The more common eloper is the *incidental* eloper. This is an individual who is drawn off the unit or out of the building. The gentleman in question demonstrated well the pattern of the incidental eloper.

His wandering pattern was observed over a two day period. Staff would place him in the lounge. His poor attention span resulted in his sitting in a chair for only a short period of time. He would soon stand and begin to wander. If anyone was behind the desk at the nurse's station located across from the lounge (diagram #4), he would be drawn to that person. He would stand at the desk for a few moments, stare at the person sitting there, lose his concentration and then continue wandering.

Even though the length of the corridors spanning the two wings created a long and valuable wandering path (diagram #4), few of the wanderers walked the east hallway.

The east hallway was hidden from view to the majority of the mentally impaired. The opening to that hall was at a sharp angle to the rest of the unit. When a mentally impaired client looked at that opening from the lounge, that person could only see a continuation of the wall. The diagram below demonstrates how the entrance to the east wing was viewed from the lounge.

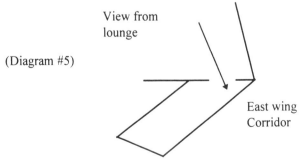

View from lounge

(Diagram #5)

East wing Corridor

The walls of the lounge and the hallways were all the same color. When the mentally impaired looked through the entrance to the east wing, they could only see a continuous wall making it obscure and oblivious from view. (Remember, *if the stimulus is not intense enough, it will be missed.*)

To assist the mentally impaired to find that part of the unit, it was necessary to paint the walls of the east wing a bright and contrasting color from the walls of the lounge and west wing. In this way the entrance would more likely stand out and the wanderers would be drawn to it, utilizing the full length of the wandering path.

THE WANDERING TOUR

The resident in question was unable to see any other corridor than the one in front of him (the west wing). This resident would turn from the nurse's station and wander down that hallway.

For this gentleman to reach the end of that hall was a major undertaking. As a mimicker he was reactive to other stimuli or *attractors.* If someone passed him heading in the opposite direction, he would turn and follow that person back down the hall. He would only tag behind until he entered the lounge, then he would trail off into that room. He was attracted by the even greater stimuli coming from the lounge - TV, people sitting, large windows to the outside. He would often wander around to each of these stimuli, then return to the nurse's station (if there was someone there), and continue down the west wing again.

His wandering pattern would finally lead him to the door at the end of the hall. On one occasion, he demonstrated well that he was an *incidental* eloper. In front of the exit door was a female resident sitting in a wheelchair. Her husband and another visitor were standing next to her carrying on a conversation. This resident walked up to the trio, stood in front of them for a few moments, turned and went back down the hall. An *aggressive* eloper would have pushed through them to get to the door.

Eventually, if not distracted, he would finally reach the door that led to the stairwell. He did not go through it immediately. Instead, he would stand in front of the door for a moment, looking at it. The door was an attractor and obviously initiated for him a thought process - "This is a door. Doors are to go through." He would then open the door. If he was noticed at this time, he could easily be returned to the unit without incident. It was obvious that he was not attempting to elope off the unit as of yet. Instead, he was being drawn through the door *looking for something familiar* and *investigating an attractor*. These are two of the basic principles involved in many of the behavioral responses by the mentally impaired elderly.

Unfortunately this unit was designed for the cognitively well, physically disabled resident. Those residents were not mobile and were restricted to a wheelchair. Therefore, there was no need for an alarm system or other security devices on the stairwell door. A cognitively well resident would not attempt the stairs in a wheelchair, but would use the elevator instead. Besides, anchored into the middle of the top step was a bar that would prevent a wheelchair from going over the first step.

ON THE WAY TO THE OUTSIDE

Once this resident walked through the exit door, he would then proceed *down the stairs*. As an aside, it is more common for the mentally impaired to go down the stairs, rather than up the stairs, for two reasons.

1) Due to the narrow or tunnel vision discussed in the previous chapter, the mentally impaired will often look down as they walk, watching the placement of their feet. Stairs going down are the first to be noticed. The stairs going up are usually not within the person's immediate visual field and are less likely taken.

2) A person experiencing progressive apraxia finds it easier to go down the stairs rather than up. To go up the stairs requires considerable strength and coordination to fight against gravity. Walking down the stairs goes with gravity, requiring less strength and coordination.

Again, if this client were stopped while going down the stairs, he could easily be returned to the unit. At this point he still did not have any thoughts of going home. It wasn't until he reached the bottom of the stairs and opened the door to the outside when he made that decision. (The only security alarms were on this door.) Once outside, he was determined he was going home, and there was no convincing him otherwise. When returned to the unit after proceeding through that exit door, he was highly aggressive for an extended period of time.

This resident became a major concern for the staff. In fact the care team was preoccupied with this gentleman. They were constantly looking for his whereabouts, making sure that he was still on the unit. Even though this resident required very little direct care, he occupied a great deal of their time. They were at a loss on how to deal with his behavior.

HIGH RISK TIMES

Staff were asked:

When is this person's worse time(s) of the day?

They identified four times of the day - meal times, shift change, late afternoon and mid evening.

1) Meal Time

On this unit the mentally impaired residents stayed in the lounge to eat their meals, and the majority of the cognitively well residents were taken to the dining room on the first floor.

At mealtimes, sixteen residents were transported down the elevator. The elevator could only accommodate four or five wheelchair clients at a time. The remainder would be positioned in front of the elevator waiting for it to return.

You will notice from the floor plan (diagram #4, page 36) that the elevator is located directly opposite the lounge. For this gentleman it was a time of highly intense stimuli. Seeing these people at the elevator became an *attractor*. It initiated the response to go with them. Each time the elevator door would open, he would attempt to get in. When staff tried to block him from entering or remove him from the elevator, he would become highly aggressive. Once he became aggressive, they would have difficulty getting him to eat his meal. The solution employed by the staff was to restrain him in a geri-chair just prior to each meal and release him from his chair at the end of the meal.

2) Shift Change

Shift change was another high risk time. At the change of shift, the day and evening staff would congregate around the nurse's station, sharing information and conversing. Then the day staff would leave the unit like a "herd of charging elephants." That stimuli also became an *attractor*. It would initiate in this client the reaction to follow either out the door or onto the elevator. When blocked or returned to the unit he would become agitated. The staff determined that it was best to confine him in a geri-chair just prior to shift change.

3) Late Afternoon

Staff identified that another high risk time was between 1630 and 1700 hours. On this unit, two staff would arrive at 1500 hours for the evening shift. One of those staff would leave the unit at 1630 hours for supper and the other would remain on the floor. At 1700 hours, the staff member on first supper break would return, two four shifts (1700 to 2100 hours) would arrive on the floor, and the other staff member would take his supper break from 1700 to 1730 hours.

Remember the schedules and routine were developed years before, when the unit predominately housed cognitively well, physically disabled residents. Those residents could be trusted not to leave the unit when only one staff member was on the floor between 1630 and 1700 hours.

The resident population changed, but the scheduling and routines remained intact. During the time when there was only one staff member on the unit, this wandering resident was at a high risk of eloping without being noticed. When the exit door alarm would sound at the bottom of the stairs between 1630 and 1700 hours, the staff member who remained on the floor was in a "damned if you do, damned if you don't" dilemma. If she left the unit to retrieve him, the other twenty-seven residents on the unit would be unattended. If she let him go, hoping staff from another unit would check the alarm, there was a chance that no one would bring him back. In either case that staff member was left with an unsafe situation. The solution employed by the care team was to restrain this gentleman in a geri-chair from 1630 to 1700 hours.

4) Mid Evening

Another high risk time was between 1830 to 2130 hours. At this time the staff were preparing residents for bed. Many of these residents were heavy care. Once they began toileting, undressing and dressing these residents, they could not be left unattended. While staff were in resident rooms performing care, they could not watch the exit door of the unit. The only time they would know that this gentleman wandered off, was when they heard the alarm to the exit door at the bottom of the stairs. They were concerned that they could not "drop everything" and run after him. They were also afraid that any delay in responding would result in their not being able to find him, or he would be injured on the busy street in front of the building. The decision was to restrain him during this time for his safety.

5) Depends Who Was On Duty

The restraint policy in this organization was poorly defined and minimally enforced. Staff were asked when else he may be restrained. They were very candid. They said that it depended which staff were on duty.

Some staff believed that if this resident needed to be restrained from 1500 to 1530 hours, he may as well remain in the chair until 1630 hours (when one staff member was left on the unit). If he was restrained until 1700 hours, he may as well remain in the chair until 1830 hours, and so on. During some evening shifts, he could be restrained in the chair for extended periods of time.

THE RESULT

A pattern has developed. This gentleman was restrained during each meal, between 1500 and 1530 hours, 1630 and 1700 hours, 1830 to

2130 hours each day. This is a mentally impaired client who has the desire to wander, who can wander, and has the energy to wander. Once he was restrained in a chair for any period of time, he would become aggressive and stay aggressive for an extended period. When aggressive, he would:

- fight all routines - toileting, bathing, dressing and undressing.
- strike other residents in the lounge when he was allowed to wander again.
- yell and swear at staff and visitors he would encounter in the hall.
- push aside residents waiting for the elevator.
- verbally be aggressive at anyone standing behind the nurse's station.
- be harder to return to the unit.

Now the rationale by some staff to restrain him for extended periods has been uncovered. It was not because they were malicious or uncaring. They believed they had valid reasons - he was aggressive whether in the chair or being returned after leaving the building. Lacking any other solution, different members of the care team justified confining him in a chair for one of the following reasons:

⇒ "He was too hard for them to handle when he was aggressive."
⇒ "They felt that it was safer for the other residents when he was confined."
⇒ "It was easier to keep track of him if he was restricted to a chair."
⇒ "It stopped him from leaving the building."
⇒ "It was more time efficient. They did not have to keep chasing him or looking where he was."

Their intervention merely substituted one problem for another. While in the chair, he would continually fight to get out, was verbally loud and abusive. When removed from the chair, he would be difficult to handle to complete any care routines. The restraining may have decreased the elopement behavior, but they now needed to find a solution for the aggressive response. It was medication.

PRESENT DAY

Before we examine the medication regime ordered for this client, it is important to summarize the sensitivity of older adults to medication. The physiological changes of aging range from individual to individual. They do not generally impact an older person's ability to maintain normal routines, but they do play a major role in medication usage. The physiological changes that can occur with aging including the following:

- decrease in the efficiency of the gastro-intestinal tract to absorb materials.
- decrease in the ability of the body to metabolize substances to break them down is lessened.
- the circulation of substances throughout the body is not as efficient.
- the body water weight of an older adult is increased.
- a lessening of lean body mass (muscle tissue).
- body fat is increased.
- a decrease in the efficiency of the liver and kidneys to excrete substances.

These changes usually occur gradually over time. This allows the older person time to become accustomed to these changes and slowly adapt to accommodate them as needed.

These physiological changes can create a sensitivity to medication that is not experienced by the younger adult. This sensitivity can result in a greater risk of adverse reactions occurring if the dosage and frequency of the medication is not adapted appropriately. More importantly, it also appears that the mentally impaired older adult may be <u>four times</u> more sensitive to certain medications than the cognitively well older adult. The reasoning behind this sensitivity is not quite clear at this time, but it is believed to be related to the biological changes occurring within the brain.

This gentleman's drug regime was as follows:

1) Lorazepam

This is an anti-anxiety agent or sedation. The standard adult dose for this medication is 2 to 4 milligrams per day. The dose for some older adults has a recommended range from 0.25 to 2 milligrams per day. This medication is addictive. If given for extended periods of time, the person must be gradually weaned off, or it could produce psychotic aggressive episodes. It should be used with caution with debilitated, elderly clients suffering from organic brain syndrome.

This gentleman was ordered one milligram, as needed (PRN), to a maximum of four times per day (QID). That did not identify how and when it was used. When the history of use was investigated further, it was noticed that he received 2 milligrams per day, every day. In the early days when the drug was first ordered, he was given 3 milligrams per day. That only occurred a few times and was never repeated.

It appears that the days he was given 3 milligrams obviously made this client quite drowsy, indicating that he could not tolerate that amount. He had been receiving 2 milligrams per day from January of the previous year to March, a total of fourteen months. In March he was taken off the drug completely. (The reason he was not taken off the drug gradually will be discussed in the next chapter.)

Initially the Lorazepam worked, but as time passed his body became more accustomed to the drug and his behavioral response intensified. (This phenomena is called the Rebound Effect and will be explained further when we discuss the Chronic Aggressive Pattern.) The dosage needed to be increased to control his aggressive behavior, but he could not tolerate any more of this drug than what he was already receiving. In November, another drug (Chlorpromazine) was ordered along with the Lorazepam to attempt to control his aggression.

2) Chlorpromazine

This is an anti-psychotic, anti-aggressive medication. It can be ordered in very large doses periodically to deal with severe aggressive behavior without creating major side effects. The standard maintenance range of dosage is 100 to 150 milligrams per day for severe cases, and 50 to 75 milligrams per day for mild cases.

This drug has a very unique side effect called tardive dyskinesia or Parkinsonian-like symptoms. Once these side effects occur, it is important to decrease the dosage or to order an anti-Parkinsonian agent. If treatment or a decrease of dosage does not occur, these Parkinsonian symptoms may continue even when the Chlorpromazine is discontinued. Tardive dyskinesia is common in elderly patients with organic brain syndrome. This gentleman was ordered 100 milligrams per day

Between November and February, the Lorazepam and Chlorpromazine were given each day. Initially that combination was tolerated by this gentleman with minimum adverse effects. As time past, he developed a gradual toxic response to these drugs, became very drowsy and experienced a dramatic loss of ability. This was the motivation to discontinue the Lorazepam in February. Once the Lorazepam was discontinued, he recovered some of his ability and responsiveness. His aggressive behavior increased in intensity as well. Unfortunately, the circumstances that caused his aggression (being restrained and leaving the building) still existed. Another drug (Diazepam) was then ordered as well.

3) Diazepam

This is an anti-anxiety agent. The dosage range of this medication is 2 to 40 milligrams per day. This drug is well known for its addictive qualities, and can have significant impact on the elderly. It is contraindicated in depression and organic brain syndrome. He was receiving 2.5 milligrams twice per day (BID) for a total of 5 milligrams per day. Unfortunately, he was still not sleeping at night. He was then ordered a sleeping pill (Restoril).

4) Restoril

The standard adult dose is 30 milligrams at bedtime. For the elderly, the dosage is recommended not to exceed 15 milligrams. This drug is to be used with caution with depression, debilitated patients and organic brain syndrome. He was receiving 30 milligrams at bedtime.

THE INTERVIEW

The interview was conducted as a final part of the assessment. During the interview, the client was asked a specific set of questions in the first few moments of the interview and then the same questions were repeated after five or six minutes (the rationale behind this will be explained later under the section on assessment). The questions were:

> How old are you?
> What year were you born?
> Who is in this picture? (Presenting a picture of family)
> What is your wife's name?

When asked these questions the first time he did not answer them. When he was shown a picture of his daughter, son-in-law and grandchildren, he did not respond either verbally or non-verbally (facial expression or gestures) that he recognized anyone in the picture.

When asked these questions again five minutes later the outcome was quite different. He was still unable to answer the first question. His response to the second question was "Nineteen, Nineteen, Nineteen, Nineteen, Nineteen, Twenty." I was not sure whether he was perseverating (uncontrollably repeating a specific word or phrase) the number nineteen and meaning to say 1919, or whether he was saying 1919, 1920. Regardless, he was correct in identifying the year he was born (1919).

He was shown the same picture of his daughter, son-in-law, and grandchildren again. This time he became somewhat distressed when he saw it. With great effort he said "Cousin, cousin, cousin, cousin." It was obvious that he had lost the names of the people in the picture, and could only call them by "cousin" (word replacement). He was aware that he was not right when he used the word "cousin." Each time he said it, he shook his head back and forth indicating no, yet he could not find another word to identify them.

He was then asked his wife's name. He said Mary (he was correct). At that point, tears were running down his cheeks. His emotional response lead to another question that I was not prepared for him to answer, "How do you feel right now?" Usually a very confused client does not have the comprehensive ability to understand the abstract meaning of this question, and is unable to answer. He responded, "I feel so alone."

On his doctor's order sheet was the order "To be restricted from all activities." The recreational activities were not geared to the mentally impaired. When this gentleman attended an inappropriate activity, he was unable to handle the stimuli, drawn to everything around him, becoming disruptive and eventually aggressive. As a result, he would usually require further sedation upon his return to the unit. It was felt that activities were "too much for him" and "it would be best to keep him from them in an attempt to lesson his aggressive outbursts, decreasing the need for sedation." (quotes from staff)

THE OVERVIEW

The assessment took place in April. The findings were as follows:

a)   It was reported by staff that he was hallucinating. This behavior began only after the Lorazepam was stopped. A possible side-effect to stopping the drug cold (psychotic behavior).

b)   He demonstrated Parkinson's symptoms - tremor lip, shuffled gait, masked expression and downcast eyes. Yet he was not given an anti-Parkinsonian agent nor was the dosage of Chlorpromazine decreased.

c)   Even though he was 75 years of age, he looked to be in his late eighties. He was quite frail, having difficulty with balance, requiring considerable energy to get out of the chair. His respirations were shallow and rapid. This change in his physical appearance had occurred only within the past six months. This was a possible result of the medications used, and the stress and exhaustion experienced.

d) He demonstrated a higher cognitive ability than anticipated, yet he was not as responsive to stimuli or direction as would be expected.

e) He showed all indications of significant depression, yet he was not receiving an anti-depressive agent (discussed under interventions).

With all of these interventions in place, the end result was that he still:

⇒ periodically wandered off the unit.
⇒ periodically left the building.
⇒ attempted to go on the elevator at meal times.
⇒ followed staff during shift change.
⇒ fought when restrained.
⇒ became aggressive.

With everything that was done, there was absolutely no change in this gentleman's behavior. Staff only focused on the client's response, not what caused it.

SUMMARY

If caring for the mentally impaired were only programming, then the solutions would be straight-forward. In actual fact, programming for the mentally impaired requires for some caregivers or even organizations, an entire re-think. This case demonstrated well the interplay of issues that contributed to the behavioral pattern presented.

a) Staff were *reactive*, waiting for the behaviors to occur before they dealt with them, rather than being *proactive*, focusing on what caused the behaviors and resolving them.

b) The environment was not conducive to meet the needs of this type of clientele. The door at the end of the hall required a security device, the elevator needed to be adapted to prevent him from using it, staff shift change needed to be subtle.

c)   Because staff were not consistent on the unit, they were unable to see the behavioral pattern, nor did they have "ownership" of the unit, feeling that they did not have any responsibility to deal with more than the day-to-day care needs.

d)   Management had not empowered staff and developed an effective team, nor prepared the organization for the transition to the present resident population.

e)   The visiting physician, responsible for this client, had minimal contact with the facility and this patient; he knew little of this individual other than what staff reported; was not trained in caring for the elderly; ordered medications as they would be ordered for a younger adult; limited authority was given to the medical director over actions of visiting physicians.

f)   Assessment tools (such as patterning, 24 hour profile, etc.) and programming options (activities, diverting, etc.) were lacking.

Some caregivers unfortunately expect the mentally impaired to be able to change or adapt to their situation, environment and the caregivers involved. The disease process and their vulnerability, the loss of recent memory and analytical ability, the range of symptomology, make that impossible. It is ourselves and what we do that must change or adapt. When we do not, the mentally impaired will communicate to us their difficulty - they will either become aggressive, wander or withdraw.

It is time now to understand the full dynamics of what leads to these responses - the Aggressive Episode, The Chronic Aggressive Pattern and The Violent Episode.

Chapter Three

THE AGGRESSIVE CYCLE

Considerable time has been spent in the previous chapters preparing for this next section - the Aggressive Cycle. We have identified the sensitivity of the mentally impaired to their living environment based on their loss of recent memory and analytical ability. When situations occur that they cannot understand, they become easily distressed. Chapter one outlined the components of the aggressive cycle.

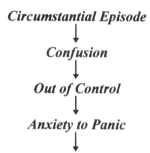

Circumstantial Episode

↓

Confusion

↓

Out of Control

↓

Anxiety to Panic

↓

Aggressive, Wandering or Withdrawn Response

Anything that confuses the mentally impaired further (called a circumstantial episode), increases their feeling of being out of control, pushes their anxiety level to a panic state, causing them to become aggressive, wander or withdraw.

This progression of events is really a crisis response employed by the mentally impaired. That response is not much different than the crisis response by any of us. When a situation is fearful and we feel out of control, we have four possible responses.

1)   Rally our energies, skills and abilities to try and solve the
       problem (*Resolve*)
2)   Fight the threat (*Fight*)

3) Run away from the threat (*Flight*)
4) Paralyzed by the threat (*Withdraw*)

A personal situation demonstrates this well.

Traveling a great deal during my speaking tours, I spend considerable time in hotels. At the end of one session, I returned to where I was staying and entered the elevator to reach my floor. A young lady entered the elevator at the same time. The standard rule in an elevator is to stare at the numbers above the door. Being still high from the seminar that day, and a seasoned traveler usually in contact with other business people of the same lifestyle, I started some small talk about the weather and the community. The other passenger responded pleasantly and pushed the button for the sixth floor. As we proceeded up, the conversation continued. It became obvious to my fellow passenger that I had not pushed a button for a floor. It just so happened that my room was also located on the sixth floor. Of course she did not know that.

She became increasingly more uncomfortable as the conversation continued and the elevator approached the sixth floor. When the elevator door opened, she scurried past me and hurried down the hall. She noticed that I was following her. My room was located down the hall past hers. The further down the hall we proceeded, the quicker her pace increased. As she reached her door, she quickly went into her room. As I walked passed, I heard every lock on that door slam shut.

I do not blame her for her actions. She did not know me or my motives. I was a possible threat to her. For her the experience was fearful, which in turn created a potential crisis situation and she responded accordingly. On the other hand, the experience gave me a great example to use for the seminar on Preventing Alzheimer's Aggression the next day.

A number of examples of distressers have been described in the previous chapters - fire drill, bus trip, activities, tour group on the unit, approaching the person to go to the bathroom, the response to my beard, etc. In each of these situations the mentally impaired were confused by what occurred around or to them. That intensified their feeling of being out of control and peaked their anxiety to a panic state.

Unfortunately when a crisis situation develops, the mentally impaired do not have the cognitive ability to resolve the situation. Their only recourse is to either fight (become aggressive), flight (wander away) or withdraw (mentally escape the distresser).

Of course the emphasis in this text is on understanding the aggressive response of the mentally impaired. The next learning priority expressed by many caregivers is to understand wandering behavior. There are few that seem to actively seek information on how to deal with the withdrawn response of the mentally impaired. The latter may be the more common response, even though it is the least investigated.

The withdrawn response of the mentally impaired is elicited when a stimuli creates intense distress, but the client does not have the physical and/or mental ability to become aggressive or wander away. This individual finds himself caught in a situation that exceeds his ability to cope. Unable to deal with the distresser in any other fashion, there is no other recourse than to become oblivious to one's surroundings in order to block out the distresser.

This may be one of the causes for the downcast eyes while sitting in a chair, falling asleep, or being totally inattentive. This is a person who is under constant stress. Eventually that stress must take its toll. In fact it may contribute to the mental, physical and emotional deterioration of the mentally impaired.

CIRCUMSTANTIAL EPISODE

A circumstantial episode is a stimuli that confuses the mentally impaired further. The disease process in combination with the Secondary Factors **makes circumstantial episodes unique to the mentally impaired elderly only**. Although other diseases not related to mental impairment (those associated with the mentally handicapped and psychiatric disorders) may have some similarities, there is <u>no other</u> disease that causes the same dynamics. The diseases associated with mental impairment create the circumstantial episodes and set the stage for the aggressive cycle. Let me explain why these qualities are unique to the mentally impaired.

It is the biological changes to the brain and the progressive deterioration in mental functioning that create the vulnerability to secondary factors (drugs, disease, approach and environment). These changes cause the circumstantial episodes by:

⇒ increasing the sensitivity of the mentally impaired to external stimuli.

⇒ creating the vulnerability to drugs and other diseases that can directly decrease existing ability.

⇒ causing the loss of ability to understand or deal with stimuli effectively.

⇒ presenting stimuli that goes beyond the person's comprehensive ability, usually being too intense or too obscure.

⇒ fragmenting past memories that results in misinterpreting present stimuli.

Likewise, it is the disease process in combination with the Secondary Factors (drugs, disease, approach, environment) that lead to the aggressive cycle by:

⇒ establishing a symptomology base (i.e. loss of recent memory, judgment, cognition, apraxia, etc.) that decreases or eliminates problem solving.

⇒ decreasing comprehensive ability, eliminating the ability to understand complex or abstract situations.

⇒ eliminating recall that would allow the person to learn how to deal differently.

⇒ impairing analytical ability that makes the person reactive to situations encountered.

⇒ combining pre-morbid personality qualities to present experiences.

$\Rightarrow$ impairing ability further, subsequently decreasing
     functioning ability further.

There are some circumstantial episodes that cannot be avoided - visitors, misinterpreted cueing, one mentally impaired client upsetting another, etc. There are others that can be controlled - approach, scheduling of activities, tours, fire drills, etc. Any of these impact on the anxiety level of the mentally impaired.

TOLERABLE ANXIETY LEVEL

Reference has been made repeatedly to the constant anxiety level of the mentally impaired. The following discussion on the Aggressive Cycle refers to that anxiety level as the *tolerable anxiety level*.

A mentally impaired client is at his *tolerable anxiety level* when he is dealing solely with the effects of the disease process. At this level he is performing at his *maximum functioning ability* based on the biological changes occurring within the brain. The term *tolerable* implies that he is void of any external distressers and his behavior or functioning ability is not influenced by any Secondary Factors (drugs, disease, approach, environment).

The term *tolerable* describes the short term effects of the disease only. In actual fact this constant anxiety level may not be tolerable over the long term. A classic text called the Nature of Stress by Hans Seyle demonstrates something of which we are all too aware - chronic stress will lead to physiological deterioration. Being under stress for an extended period of time impacts on energy level, sleep pattern, digestion, and emotional state. If stress occurs too long without substantial relief, then it can also lead to high blood pressure, ulcers, etc.

The mentally impaired are under constant stress. Every noise, face, stimuli has to be continuously analyzed. The example in chapter one that simulated admission to long term care demonstrates this stress well. In that simulation you were to imagine being blindfolded with ear plugs placed in your ears and then moved to a location you did not know. The stress that prolonged experience creates can only be tolerated for so long before it takes its toll. The daily physical, emotional and mental investment by this clientele can only lead to exhaustion and physical and mental deterioration.

In fact this exhaustion becomes one of the thirty-two causes of aggression discussed in the next chapter. Physical and mental exhaustion are two of the reasons for the change in behavior and functioning ability of some mentally impaired on a daily basis. Some are more able to complete certain tasks in the morning when they are well rested, than in the evening when they are tired. Likewise, some things are better tolerated early in the day, but those same things become distressers later in the day.

Imagine the impact of that stress daily for the rest of one's life. It is no wonder that the mentally impaired are sensitive to any added stimuli or pressure.

We have now defined this individual's vulnerability, the relationship between the disease process and Secondary Factors, circumstantial episodes, tolerable anxiety level, and maximum performance level. All of these in combination create the aggressive cycle which creates the Aggressive Episode, the Chronic Aggressive Pattern and the Violent Episode.

THE AGGRESSIVE EPISODE

(Diagram #6)

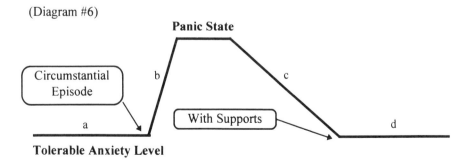

When a circumstantial episode occurs (such as a fire drill) the client becomes confused by the noise and commotion it creates. That

57

immediately increases her feeling of being out of control. Her anxiety level (*line 'a', diagram #6*) is pushed to a panic state (*line 'b'*). The client becomes loud and vocal as a result.

If the environment or programming is supportive and the needed intervention strategies to decrease the distresser are employed - divert, re-direct or back off (to be discussed in detail later), then in time (*line 'c'*) she will return to her tolerable anxiety level (*line 'd'*).

It is important to emphasize the difference between the line that leads up to the panic state and the line that goes down from it. The impact of the circumstantial episode is immediate (*line 'b'*). After the panic state the line has a gradual decline (*line 'c'*). This represents the amount of time required for the client to settle and return to her tolerable anxiety level and maximum functioning ability. Of course the angle of that line or the amount of time required is individualized. It depends on many factors: the intensity and type of stimuli, the physical state of the client, the symptomology, past history of stress response, the location, the people around, etc. The drop from panic state to tolerable anxiety level rarely occurs quickly. In fact for some it may require many hours.

When the aggressive cycle is compared to the original graph presented in chapter one, it demonstrates in a smaller scale what occurs when a Secondary Factor is encountered.

(Diagram #7)

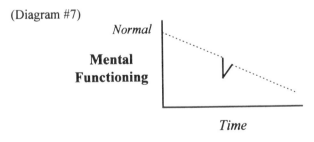

The dotted line represents the disease process. The solid line represents the impact of this secondary factor and the resultant impact on ability and subsequent behavior. Of course the time frame is condensed to show the effect.

This response to circumstantial episodes is normal with the mentally impaired and cannot be avoided. The need to set the supports to deal with repeated distressers is a commonplace occurrence. Once the response does occur, then the caregiver's responsibility is to *investigate* what may have caused it (utilizing a series of functional assessment tools such as patterning) to be able to help this person avoid the same response in the future. As will be discussed, the skilled *investigative* caregiver over time will learn to identify the preemptive cueing that will allow her to prevent the client from going into a panic state in the first place.

The problem occurs when the behavior does not initiate a different response by the caregiver. Either the freedom or willingness to adapt the care routine and supports is not in place, or the strategies to resolve the situation are not implemented. Instead the behavioral response is ignored, and the care routine is maintained. That then leads to the Chronic Aggressive Pattern.

THE CHRONIC AGGRESSIVE PATTERN

(Diagram #8)

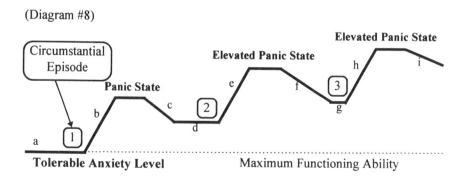

Again the fire alarm sounds (circumstantial episode #1). This client becomes confused by the noise and commotion. She feels further out of control, her anxiety is peaked to a panic state. She becomes loud and verbal in response. Unfortunately the supports are not in place - divert, re-direct or back off and the demands placed upon the client are not adjusted. Even before she returns to her tolerable anxiety level (*line 'a'*), she is taken for a tub bath not fifteen minutes after the fire drill.

Normally this individual does not have a problem with her bath. Unfortunately, when the bath is introduced at a time when her anxiety level is already elevated, she cannot handle the added pressure. A stimuli is initiated when she is hypersensitive and her tolerance has decreased. This will only intensify her feeling of being out of control.

She may still go to the tub, but she will be resistive (pulling away), loud and verbal throughout the entire procedure. She may even require two staff rather than one to get her into the tub and complete the bath. Likewise, tasks she was able to complete independently when at her maximum functioning level (i.e. washing her face and hands during the bath, etc.) may be lost. She is too distracted by what is occurring around and to her, making it difficult to concentrate on the task at hand.

Her resistive movements during her bath (pulling away, blocking staff from washing her, etc.) results in staff accidentally getting soap in her eyes. That event now becomes another circumstantial episode (#2). She cannot understand the stinging sensation experienced. Her anxiety is peaked again, but this time to an even higher panic state. She is not only resistive, loud and verbal, but also swearing. Examine the graph to identify what has occurred.

1) The bath was introduced before her anxiety level returned to its tolerable state (*line 'd'*). This is a time when she is hypersensitive to stimuli. The "soap in her eyes" becomes the second circumstantial episode (#2).

2) The panic state occurring from the second circumstantial episode is higher than the panic state from the first. This represents the increased feeling of being out of control and intensified confusion. It is important to note that the soap in her eyes that created the second circumstantial episode (#2), would probably have been a circumstantial episode had there not been a fire drill. Had this event occurred in isolation, it would have resulted in her being loud and verbal. Now it occurred in conjunction with the response to the fire drill, intensifying her response.

3) Compare the lines that lead down from the panic state after each event (*line 'c'* and *'f'*). You will notice that *line 'f'* is at a more gradual decline. This illustrates that the combined impact of the first and second circumstantial episode takes longer for her to return to her tolerable anxiety level. Her elevated emotional state suggests that:

- certain diversional or re-directing strategies that could have been successful after the first circumstantial episode (line 'c') may not work now.

or

- she will require a longer time left alone in order for her to return to her tolerable anxiety state than after the first circumstantial episode.

If the supports are still not initiated, and the care routine is continued, it will lead to a further acceleration of events. For example, a half an hour after her bath she is taken to lunch.

During meals the person sitting next to her (who is also mentally impaired), usually reaches for this client's food. Under normal circumstances, when this client is at her tolerable anxiety level (*line a*), she has no problem with his actions. She just takes his hand and pushes it aside. When he attempts to steal her food during this meal, when she is hypersensitive to stimuli, her response is very different. It now becomes a circumstantial episode (#3). She is loud, verbal, and swearing, but now also slapping at anyone who comes near and she then refuses to eat. The results are diagrammatically represented in the graph (diagram #8, page 59).

1) Lunch was introduced when she was hypersensitive to stimuli (*line 'f'*). What before was tolerated and had no effect on behavior or functioning ability, now becomes a circumstantial episode, initiating a panic state.

2) Furthermore her panic state is elevated higher than the previous response. The third circumstantial episode places her further out of control, requiring her response to match the emotional intensity experienced. Her response increases in severity as a result.

3) Compare *line 'a'*, with *line 'd'* and *'g'*. The length of each line is shorter. The first line (*a*), demonstrates that the first circumstantial episode may take considerable time to develop. At this point the client's tolerance level to stimuli is at its greatest intensity. The next line (*d*) demonstrates that the occurrence of the second circumstantial episode is much quicker than the first. The third line (*g*) demonstrates that the incidence for the third circumstantial episode occurs even more quickly. The reason for the shortening of these lines is that as each event occurs, the client's tolerance to further stimuli is lessened.

4) Comparing the lines descending from the panic state also shows a marked difference. *Line 'f'* has a more gradual decline from *line 'c'*, and *line 'i'* an even more gradual incline than *line 'f'*. This demonstrates the increased time it takes for the client to return to her tolerable anxiety level. At this time many of the diversional or re-directing strategies that would normally be effective to decrease this client's emotional state, will be less effective. She may now be limited to responding favorably to only a few intervention strategies. She would definitely need to be left alone for a considerable period of time to show any marked decrease in her distress level.

If the caregiver does not employ the necessary or appropriate intervention strategies at this time, then all this can only progress to the next level - a Violent Episode.

THE VIOLENT EPISODE

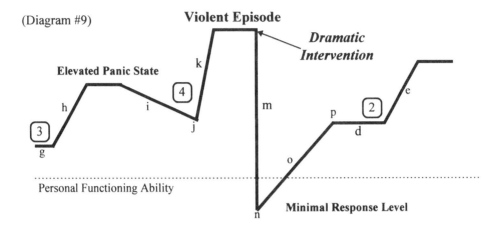

(Diagram #9)

The aggressive cycle has progressed - from the fire drill, to soap in her eyes during the tub bath, to another mentally impaired resident stealing her food during mealtime. She is just beginning to settle after the altercation in the dining room (*line 'i'*). Staff inappropriately assess that the best thing for her is to attend her favorite recreational activity, believing that this will be an effective distracter and change her behavior.

This person needs to only be in a room with a few people (*point 'j'*), and she will lose control again. This time she is not only loud, verbal and swearing, but also physically violent. She is striking out at everyone near her. At this time there is a need for dramatic intervention. She will be heavily sedated. Again return to the graph (diagram #9).

1) Her favorite recreational activity was introduced at a point of intense hypersensitivity to any further stimuli (*line 'i'*). It now becomes a circumstantial episode. This represents a significant progression of events.

63

- The fire drill and soap in her eyes during the bath were obvious circumstantial episodes. The possibility for any mentally impaired client to deal with either of these effectively is minimal.
- The other client attempting to steal her food should have been a circumstantial episode. Under normal circumstances, when this client is at her tolerable anxiety level, she is able to tolerate his actions. Once her sensitivity was increased, this event became a circumstantial episode.
- In the example that created the Violent Episode, an event that normally elicits positive feelings with this client and has been successfully used as a diversional tactic in the past to change behavior, has become a circumstantial episode.

This demonstrates a significant concept: *As the anxiety level of the mentally impaired is elevated, what previously was not a circumstantial episode becomes one. As it intensifies further, the potential for all stimuli to become circumstantial episodes occurs.*

2) Her reaction to this stimuli (the activity) is immediate (*point 'j'*). Unlike the previous circumstantial episodes, it takes no time for her to feel pressured, out of control and her already peaked anxiety state to elevate to a violent response (*line 'k'*).

3) The Violent Response is a point where the client's emotional state has eliminated all existing functioning ability. Strengths or previous abilities have been negated. Tolerance is non-existent. The person is totally overwhelmed by the experience and is in a *defensive response* to eliminate the pressures encountered.

4) The dramatic intervention employed when she is violent also has an immediate effect (*line 'm'*). The problem with the type and amount of sedation needed is that it does not return her to her tolerable anxiety level, but drags her well below her

maximum functioning ability (*point 'n'*). She is now heavily sedated, and has no energy to get out of the chair or complete any task. She is drowsy, which dulls her cognitive ability, making it difficult to respond to even basic stimuli.

5) Being heavily sedated does not allow the person to go from being sedated to not being sedated. There is a significant recovery time (*line 'o'*). As she recovers from the sedation, she does not return to her tolerable anxiety level, but at a higher level of anxiety (*point 'p'*). During this time she is less able to analyze stimuli, her reaction time is slower and her endurance has been lessened. At *point 'p'* her sensitivity is increased and her tolerance level decreased. In essence she as coming out of the sedation at the same level that created the second circumstantial episode (*line 'd'*), or even higher. She is primed for the pattern to begin again.

THE TOO COMMON INTERVENTION STRATEGY

The most common request for assistance by many caregivers is when a mentally impaired client becomes physically violent. Requesting intervention strategies at this time is too late. There is little that can be done when a person is violent except to sedate, restrain and/or back off. Neither of these is successful, and as demonstrated in the case study in chapter two, they can be detrimental to the individual.

Waiting for a mentally impaired client to reach this severity of response results in crisis intervention. Crisis intervention is a reactive process - it involves allowing an event to occur to create the behavioral response, then being forced to implement a dramatic course of action to resolve it. This is considered a passive care focus that not only is ineffective, but will also accelerate the incidence of violent episodes.

To demonstrate this point we need only review the case example in Chapter Two. Lorazepam was given to deal with the violent behavior caused by being restrained in the chair or returned after leaving the building. When given the drug, it initially had the desired sedating effect. It decreased his energy level and awareness to his surroundings.

It was adequate enough to subdue his behavior and the violent episodes decreased in severity, but not necessarily in frequency.

As time passed, his body became more acclimatized to the medication. This meant that his energy level and awareness to his surroundings increased somewhat. Unfortunately, the same distressers still existed (being restrained and leaving the building). As the efficiency of the drug decreased, it created a *rebound effect* and contributed to the increased severity of his violent behavior.

The rebound effect occurs
when the effectiveness of the medication decreases,
the causative factor is not removed,
leaving the client to revert back to the original behavior
with greater frequency and intensity.

Before receiving the Lorazepam, his cognitive abilities and skills allowed him to cope well with a variety of stimuli - care routine, visitors, other residents in the lounge, etc. Initially these did not create distressers or illicit the aggressive cycle. Unfortunately, in order for the Lorazepam to control his violent behavior, it also dulled his cognitive skills and decreased his functioning ability. It made the client more hypersensitive and less tolerable to stimuli while under the influence of the medication than without it.

As the initial effects of the drug lost some of its potency, his awareness of his surroundings and his energy level increased. As his awareness increased, he was less able to handle the stimuli encountered (care routines, visitors, other residents, etc.) and these became circumstantial episodes. As his energy level increased, he became violent more quickly with less provocation. The fact remains -

When the causative factors that initiated the behavior
are not controlled or removed,
the need is always for a higher dosage of medication.

Medication as a treatment modality is always limited by the sensitivity of the mentally impaired to the drugs commonly used. Usually the maximum dose is reached before the behavior is totally subdued. Administering any more of that specific drug would only cause a toxic response and have dire consequences. This requires another medication in addition to the first to control the behavioral response. The consequence becomes a teeter-totter effect of medication dispensing and response:

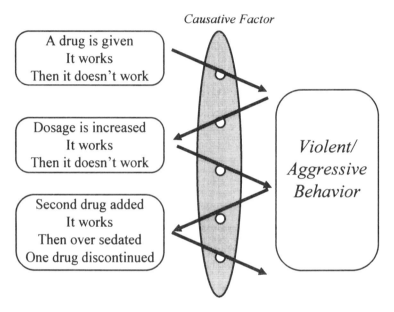

Causative Factor

A drug is given
It works
Then it doesn't work

Dosage is increased
It works
Then it doesn't work

Second drug added
It works
Then over sedated
One drug discontinued

*Violent/
Aggressive
Behavior*

The pattern is continued until eventually there is no further need for sedation. The physical deterioration created by this drug regime will probably result in the client losing a majority of physical and mental abilities. At some point this person will become non-ambulatory, non-communicative, and non-responsive - total care.

Focusing on the violent episode is employing the intervention at the wrong time. Working effectively with the mentally impaired is not intervening after a Violent Episode, it is intervening at the first Aggressive Episode. This requires the care focus to be proactive - dealing with the behavior before it occurs. This can only be achieved by an *investigative* caregiver - one who is successful at *Preventing Alzheimer's Aggression.*

IN DEFENSE OF THE PHYSICIAN

In the previous case (Chapter Two) the most common criticism is leveled at the physician. There is no doubt that the physician in question required more knowledge of medication use in the elderly and that the medical director required more authority to challenge visiting physicians who are not practicing based on the needs of the clients. But it is time to set the record straight. The physician was only caught in the care dynamics that existed. An important question must be asked.

Who orders medication for the mentally impaired older client?

The physician may write the order, but he is often influenced by the staff performing the care. If a long term care organization experiences any of the following:

- Limited training in caring for the mentally impaired elderly.
- A lack of appropriate programming for this clientele.
- Employing intervention strategies that worked well with the cognitively well.
- An environmental design geared for the cognitively well.
- Minimal behavioral and functional assessment tools.
- Out-dated care routines.
- Limited empowering of staff.

Then the outcome is predictable - aggressive/violent episodes by the mentally impaired will be a common place occurrence, and medication will be the primary intervention strategy employed.

Let me outline a scenario that has been presented to thousands of caregivers during my seminars. They have commented repeatedly that it best describes one of the frustrations they frequently encounter. Imagine the following:

A long term care facility that has specialized in caring for the cognitively well, physically disabled client, where:

- the majority of part time staff (both registered nurses and direct line staff) are not consistently assigned to a specific unit. Instead they float the building, moving from unit to unit.
- a unit has been set aside to house the mentally impaired residents, but there is no programming formally arranged.
- the registered nursing staff are not formally trained as managers, and the role of managing is not clearly defined.
- there is poor communication and linkage between care teams from shift to shift.
- the visiting physicians are not active members of the care team.

In this facility, the full time registered nurse who normally works the unit housing the mentally impaired resident is:

- a skilled nurse.
- effective at problem solving and ensuring accountability of staff performance.
- understands the need of the mentally impaired.
- has a working knowledge of programming strategies.

The few staff who work consistently on her unit have had limited formal training on caring for the mentally impaired, but:

- instinctively work well with this clientele.
- are supportive in their approach.
- provide as much time as possible when completing tasks.
- are flexible, willing to adapt their routine depending on the needs of the individual at that time.
- have learned skills that allow them to decrease the agitation of the mentally impaired before it accelerates to a Violent Episode.

The resident in question is mentally impaired and highly sensitive to stimuli. This resident encounters the fire drill. When the registered nurse and direct line staff described above are on duty, they effectively decrease her agitation and help her to settle. The matter progresses no further. These next two days, these staff are off duty. Replacing them is the following.

A part time registered nurse is now in charge of the unit for the next two days. She is:

- a skilled nurse.
- works only two days a week, frequently assigned to different units.
- feels no ownership for any one unit.
- does not clearly understand the needs of mentally impaired.
- is not familiar with programming options for this clientele.

The replacement direct line staff are either part time or float staff who work the entire building. They:

- feel no ownership for any one unit.
- do not know the specific idiosyncrasies of the residents on this unit.
- have not been trained to care for the mentally impaired.
- do not understand their behavior or the strategies to defuse it.
- focus primarily on the duties and tasks to be completed for the shift assigned.

They encounter the same resident who is highly sensitive to stimuli. The fire drill sounds, the resident becomes loud and verbal. These staff do not respond to her behavioral change. They instead take her for her assigned tub bath. She gets soap in her eyes, is loud, verbal and swearing. They then take her for lunch. Another resident attempts to steal her food, she is loud, verbal, swearing and slapping. They know from the chart that she enjoys a specific recreational activity and feel that this might be the best for her. During the activity, the resident becomes violent.

At a loss of what to do, they approach the part time registered nurse stating, "You had better do something about this lady. She is going to hurt somebody." The doctor arrives on the unit. He asks the part time registered nurse, "Are there any problems?" The nurse says, "Yes, you had better order something for this lady. She has been violent."

Is it realistic to ask the physician how to care for a mentally impaired older client? There are few doctors who have worked with this clientele eight hours per day for an extended period of time. That is not a criticism of the physician's ability. Unless that physician is a specialist in the field, knows the full dynamics of what is occurring, not only with the resident but also on the unit and has the authority and time to make change, he will be stymied. He cannot come up with an alternate strategy when the person is violent, but he is placed in the position where action must be taken. He must provide a solution or be held accountable if the resident injures someone else. The physician will often ask, "What do you want?"

The registered nurse may respond, "Haldol (sedation)." The physician, not knowing the client and concerned about the dosage, may state, "Haldol 0.5 milligrams." The registered nurse concerned about the intensity of the violent behavior and the safety of all around may respond back, "I don't think that will be enough, she is terribly upset." The physicians response, "All right Haldol 1.0 milligram."

The full time registered nurse and direct line staff return to the unit after their two days off duty. They find this client sedated.

We have finally identified one of the greatest challenges in working with the mentally impaired elderly - it is the conflict between those who *think they know* how to care for the mentally impaired versus those who *really know.*

Those who think they know see medication as their first choice.
Those who really know see medication as their last choice.

Unless this conflict is resolved, it is the mentally impaired client who will suffer the consequences.

SUMMARY

Programming for the mentally impaired is not just a group of strategies implemented to resolve a problem. It is a combination of events that must work in unison to have the desired result. The programming options of the next chapters are valuable, but they can only be totally effective when the following objectives are met.

1) Provide security and safety for the wandering client.
2) Provide the mentally impaired with consistency in routines and staff.
3) Establish a philosophy specific to the needs of the mentally impaired.
4) Have a specific care process that involves analysis and assessment of cognitive functioning, with an admission and discharge procedure for a specialized unit.
5) Have available specific social and activity programs geared to cognitive functioning level.
6) Have staff skilled in working with the mentally impaired in the area of: approach, communication, assessment and understanding.
7) Have a mechanism to define the individual vulnerability of each client.
8) Have an environment that is adapted to the needs of the clientele.

These are the objectives of Supportive Therapy* (outlined in detail in the text The Tactics of Supportive Therapy). They reflect the sensitivity of this clientele, and the challenges of the specialty. Patchwork solutions will have short term gains. Focusing on the needs of the care environment in which this person is exposed is the key to success. Remember the two basic concepts defined in chapter one.

> *Symptoms caused by the disease cannot be stopped, only made tolerable*

> *If a symptom of an Alzheimer's victim can be stopped with something other than medication, then it is not Alzheimer's that is causing it.*

We have finally disclosed the underlying theme of this text. The focus of care is not "how do we change the mentally impaired to deal differently with what we do." It is **how do we change ourselves and how we perform our care to meet the specific needs of the individual**. Once that is accepted and consistent by all who care for this clientele, then and only then can we possibly prevent aggressive behavior of the mentally impaired from occurring.

It is time now to define *programming* as it relates to aggressive behavior.

[*Note: Refer to the questionnaire "Evaluating The Care Process for the Mentally Impaired Elderly" Chapter Seven, the *Tactics of Supportive Therapy*. This is a multi-paged questionnaire used to evaluate how effective an organization is in achieving these objectives.]

Chapter Four

32 CAUSES OF AGGRESSION

Imagine the following:

A cognitively well older client
Has experienced a stroke/
Total paralysis on the *right* side of her body
She is unable to move her right arm or leg/

While lying in bed
Her breakfast is always placed on a bedside table to the *right* of
    her
The right bedside rail is up/
In order to eat her meal
She must reach over the right side of her body/
This requires considerable concentration to perform the task
She takes more time and energy than would be necessary if the
    tray were located on her left side/

The inappropriate location of her tray occurs at every meal
Three times per day, every day/
The way the meal is served is stressful and exhausting for her/
She never complains
She never becomes angry
She just *struggles* with what needs to be done/

Staff watch her each time/
They do not alter the location of her meal
They do not respond to her obvious frustration
Or assist in any way/
They maintain the same pattern regardless of her need/

To watch an individual such as this unduly struggle with her meal would spark someone to ask, "Why are the caregivers doing that?" She requires things to be placed closest to her left side. Even though she is able to do the task, it is inappropriate given her limitations and abilities. If it is necessary to wait for her to become visibly angry in order to change the situation, then someone must question the assessment ability of the caregiver to meet this person's needs with such a simple task.

This scenario depicts well the "not so obvious" experiences of the mentally impaired. Their symptoms are not as visible as a paralyzed right side. If it is necessary to wait for the mentally impaired to blatantly show aggressive or violent behavior before something is done, then we have failed this individual. The challenge in working with the mentally impaired is that their ability to communicate may be more subtle then blatant aggressive behavior. However, the mentally impaired *always* do communicate. If we are capable of reading the behavioral cueing, then we will be successful in preventing Alzheimer's aggression from occurring.

LEVELS OF AGGRESSION

In the previous discussions we have referred to different types and intensities of aggressive behavior. In actual fact the aggressive response can be divided into three levels:

> ⇒ *Resistive Response*
> ⇒ *Aggressive Response*
> ⇒ *Violent Response*

The Resistive Response represents a *pulling away*. It can be identified by the following cues:

> ⇒ comments - these involve a variety of phrases to indicate that the individual is distressed by what is occurring around or to him. Examples could include, "Leave me alone." "I don't want to." "Help, she is hurting me." "Where is my daughter?" (summoning for help)

⇒ actions - these involve a variety of mannerisms, expressions or physical movements such as pulling hands back, holding on to individuals or objects, wandering, wide eyed fearful facial expression, etc.

The Aggressive Response is a *pushing away*. It is a more intensified response that can be identified by:

⇒ comments - these are much more forceful (increased volume and harsher tone), including intimidating words (swearing) or phrases such as "Get out of here." "I won't do that." "I'll get you for that."

⇒ actions - these involve more forceful physical actions, mannerisms and expressions such as pushing, intimating posture, slapping, scratching, head butting, etc.

The Violent Response is a crisis response. As identified in the previous chapter, it is a defense reaction. This is an individual who can no longer handle the stresser encountered and is lashing out in order to defend himself from what is happening. The demands or circumstances have exceeded his abilities. This person is in a crisis state. His comments and actions will be extreme, and result in the person destroying objects or injuring others around him. At this point dramatic intervention normally needs to be employed to resolve the situation.

In actual fact these levels are not independent. A stressful situation will normally begin with a resistive response. If the stresser is not removed or decreased, then it will lead to an aggressive response. Again, if it is not dealt with, it will lead to a violent response. Hence the basis for the aggressive cycle.

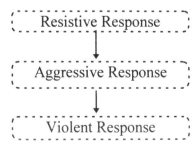

Highly Individualized Behavior

Aggression is a highly complex, personalized emotion. One's outward response cannot be the only measuring tool to define the intensity of the stress creating it. In actual fact:

⇒ some mentally impaired do not have the ability to become aggressive or violent.

⇒ others take considerable time to be pushed to an aggressive state, with warning cues always present.

⇒ others will immediately snap into a violent response over what seems to be the simplest stimuli.

Many believe that the more intense the behavioral reaction, the more intense the distresser causing it. In fact that may not be accurate. The person who is demonstrating a resistive response may be experiencing as an intense a distress situation, but is simply unable to communicate it in a violent manner. This demonstrates that:

The intensity of the stresser
may not be in direct proportion
to the intensity of the response.

Each mentally impaired client will have a different way of reacting to any given distresser.

- The majority will experience a progression in emotional intensity in the exact manner as was described by the graphs of the Aggressive Cycle.
- Some mentally impaired will immediately react to stimuli with an aggressive or even violent response as soon as the distresser is encountered. The graph described in the previous chapter peaks quickly to an intense aggressive response or even a violent episode. This is an individual with a low tolerance level and a quick reaction time.
- Others will experience a progression of emotional build-up under most circumstances, as defined by the graph. However specific people or events will create an abnormally intense

aggressive or even violent response (example presented in the opening of the text where the client reacted to my beard and threw the vase).

- Some mentally impaired clients do not have the personal make-up or cognitive and/or mental ability to become violent, leaving the aggressive response as their maximum behavioral reaction.
- Others do not have the personal make-up or cognitive and/or mental ability to become aggressive, leaving the resistive response as the greatest intensity that will be experienced.

The reaction by the caregiver to these varieties of response is what exposes the care philosophy of any setting, and the intervention and programming strategies that may be employed. To understand this further, it is important to distinguish between a care setting with a *passive care focus* from one with a *quality care focus*.

A setting that has not adapted its philosophy and care to the specific needs of the mentally impaired client usually has a *passive care focus*. In this type of care environment, it appears that the primary motivation to intervene is when the staff experience a client behavior that *they* cannot handle. This often creates care oriented rather than client centered programming.

In a passive care focus, something has to happen to motivate the care team into action - a client is out of control, injuring someone, fighting care routines, etc. In this environment, the caregiver often misses or ignores the subtle cues demonstrated by a mentally impaired client. The caregiver's response is reactive - responding only to situations that are the most difficult to resolve (a violent episode). Unfortunately, the needs of the mentally impaired who are unable to present obvious aggressive or violent behavior are often overlooked.

A *quality care focused* environment has a much different philosophy. It is truly client centered, using the client's behavior as a part of their assessment process. The caregiver in this setting continuously investigates potential stressors regardless of the intensity of the behavioral response of the client. This is a setting that is proactive or preventative in nature. In fact, it is unusual for staff in this setting to encounter intense aggressive behavior, let alone violent episodes from their clients.

What is ironic is that the former approach is intended to simplify the care routine in order to decrease staff stress. The latter approach is attempting to adapt their care routine in order to decrease client stress. However, it is the latter approach that is more successful in decreasing work load and job related stress for staff than the former. Let me explain.

NORMAL BEHAVIOR

The major difference between a quality care setting and a passive one is based on the expectations the caregivers have about the clientele. The care team of a quality care setting know that resistive/aggressive behavior of the mentally impaired is normal behavior, and physical violence is not.

Imagine:

> You are mentally impaired
> Sitting in a chair
> You want to stay in that chair/
>
> You cannot communicate what you want/
> Either you have *disjointed thought*
> Where you cannot keep your thoughts in order
> Long enough to construct a sentence/
> Or you have lost so much vocabulary
> That you do not have enough words to complete a sentence/
> Either way, you cannot verbally express what you want/
>
> I approach you and try to get you to stand from the chair/
> What would be your response?

You would resist me. That is normal behavior for the mentally impaired - how else can someone communicate what they want or don't want when they cannot communicate verbally? When such a response is encountered, it requires the caregiver to alter her approach and/or use specific strategies to draw you from the chair, or back off until you are more receptive.

Those from a passive care setting who do not understand the mentally impaired respond differently to what is experienced.

- Some wrongly misinterpret resistive behavior as "aggression," and demand a more dramatic intervention (often medication) because the person is not cooperative with the scheduled *task*.

- Others will ignore the behavior in order to complete the *task*, accelerating the client to an aggressive response, or even a violent episode, also requiring medication intervention.

It is easy to see the common denominator in these two scenarios - it is the "task." The client in a passive care setting is expected and required to adapt to the care routine. The care dynamics appear as follows:

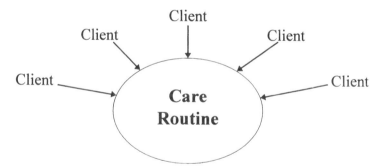

In this setting the care routine is scheduled - bathing, mealtime, activities, etc. - and the mentally impaired are expected to perform those tasks at the defined times. Change in the routine or other intervention strategies (usually medication) is only considered when the client blocks the scheduled task by an intense aggressive or violent response. In that case, the caregiver sees the client as the "problem," not the care routine, approach, environment, etc. In this setting, the staff are care oriented rather than client centered.

Yet in that same setting, staff who work with the cognitively well, physically disabled client do not wait for a decubitis ulcer (skin breakdown) to occur before preventative measures are taken. They begin treatment with any reddened area. During bathing or back massage, they *adjust* their normal routine to focus more on that vulnerable location in hopes of preventing skin breakdown from ever occurring. They read the subtle cues and employ the necessary preventative measures. That is considered quality care.

The approach of a quality care setting for the mentally impaired takes on a similar focus. Investigative caregivers are successful because of their greater receptivity to the behavioral responses of the mentally impaired. They use this client's behavior not as something that should be avoided, but as a marker or cue to indicate there may be a problem and a subsequent need to adjust what is being done. They view the care routine in a somewhat different manner:

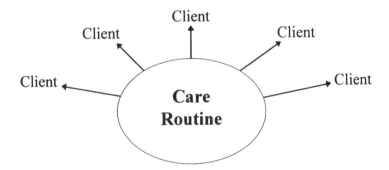

They know that they are more effective when the care routine is adjusted to fit the individual client, rather than attempting to make the client fit the care routine. They possess the key quality of programming that ensures success - they are flexible in what they do and how they do it.

Some will legitimately say - "There are times when you can't leave the person just because she is uncooperative. Certain things have to be done." The reality of working with this clientele is that there are times when nothing will work (divert, re-direct or back away) and you just have "to do." When a client has become incontinent, she cannot be allowed to remain in that state indefinitely just because she does not want to change her clothes. The fact is that she has to be changed.

However, "doing" for the sake of doing, or "doing" and being sensitive to the clientele can create different outcomes.

In a passive care setting she will be changed, because achieving that will be the primary focus of the care team. However, in a quality care setting, the primary focus of the staff will be to decrease the distress created by changing her. They adapt what they need to do to this individual's ability and vulnerability.

Let us parallel these two settings to see the difference:

Quality Care Setting	Passive Care Setting
1) Whoever changes her would be the caregiver on duty who has the greatest rapport.	1) Whoever is assigned to her or discovers her will complete the task regardless of the relationship that exists.
2) Staff will know the specific diverting or distracting tactics that are successful with this client. They are employed before, during and after the event.	2) The approach will be done with limited, general or even no diverting or distracting tactics employed. The tactics will not be defined, communicated to all staff, or not learned by the specific caregiver.
3) After it is over, the care team will "back off" completely on all other avenues of the care routine until she settles - including meals, activities, etc.	3) After it is over, the care routine will continue as scheduled regardless of her response to being changed.
4) Through the time she is stressed, the caregiver will make periodic contact, continually employing diverting or distracting techniques knowing that as she is settling she is more receptive, and these will also further hasten her returning to her "normal" state.	4) Her emotional state will escalate and functioning ability decrease. She will likely be sedated if the behavior intensifies to a great enough response.

The one on the left results in no further escalating to a more intense behavioral response. The one to the right has all the trappings of the Aggressive Cycle.

To this point the emphasis in understanding aggressive behavior has been on the philosophy and focus of the care process. Before assessment tools and programming options can be considered, a detailed understanding of what causes aggressive behavior with the mentally impaired must be established.

THE 32 CAUSES OF AGGRESSION

The following is the list of *32 causes of aggressive behavior* and a brief description of how they apply to the mentally impaired. The goal at this point is to set the foundation for the assessment tools and programming options that will be discussed in detail in the next two chapters. The causes that have been addressed in the previous chapters and those that are described in detail in the text the Tactics of Supportive Therapy have only been summarized in this section.

Remember that each of these causes are not characteristic to all mentally impaired clients. Since the needs, symptomology and vulnerability of each mentally impaired client is individualized, the causative factors that can lead to aggression are also individualized. Once the causes have been defined, we can then discuss the necessary assessment tools that will disclose which applies to each client.

1) *Depression*

It has been estimated that at least 75% of those who are mentally impaired have a significant degree of depression. In fact that number may be low. Suggesting that depression is associated with mental impairment is understandable. A mentally impaired client may not know exactly what he has lost, but there is often this constant foreboding that something is missing, hence the behavior of "looking for something familiar."

Depression only complicates the disease further. The symptoms of depression - loss of energy, apathy, poor self image, etc. can lessen receptivity to any task. Often when depression is suspected, it is treated with anti-depressive medication. The standard five to six weeks of administration to determine its effectiveness may not be appropriate for the mentally impaired elderly. They may require a longer time period on the drug before any change is noted. If there is no noted mood elevation in the appropriate time that the drug should be dispensed, then it is commonly discontinued.

By the way, when an anti-depressive agent is effective, there may be an increase in aggressive behavior. When depressed, energy levels wane and a person withdraws, decreasing awareness to his surroundings. When an anti-depressive drug is effective, it improves all of those areas, increasing a person's sensitivity to his surroundings and elevating his reactive ability. If the stressors causing the aggressive response are not removed, the behavior may only intensify.

2) *Time*

The problem with the mentally impaired and time is that time changes every minute. The mentally impaired cannot recall a stationary point from which to measure time passage. If they are able to recall anything, it will only be events. It is easy to understand the confusion this creates when a caregiver states, "It is time to eat (lunch)." This client will often respond, "I just ate." The person does not remember that it was four hours ago at breakfast. Or when someone says, "Time to have your bath," the client's response in this case will be, "I just had one." Agreed, but that was a week ago.

When time passage is lost but events can still be recalled, it creates the potential for conflict, and fertile grounds for an aggressive response.

3) *Timing*

With some mentally impaired it is better to perform intimate and complex care like a bath in the morning when they are well rested than in the evening when they are tired. When tired, their tolerance level to stimuli is decreased and their patience to meet the demands of the task at hand are lessened.

On the other hand, in some cases it is better to perform intimate and complex care such as a bath in the evening when the person is tired, than in the morning when she is rested. In the morning the person's cognitive ability is greater, making the individual more sensitive to stimuli. Likewise in the morning the person has the energy level to fight the procedure. In the evening, when the person is tired, her cognitive and physical abilities have decreased, making her less sensitive to the stimuli and less apt to fight the procedure.

4) *Approach*

We have demonstrated on frequent occasions that at times our actions are faster than the person's ability to analyze them. This implies that the caregiver may at times be the cause of aggression. The pitfalls in approaching the mentally impaired will be discussed in detail in chapter seven.

5) *Word Comprehension*

This was presented in chapter two. Some mentally impaired know the object but cannot understand the word. Others know the word but cannot understand the object. When these are not addressed, the person will be easily confused about what is being asked, and potentially respond in an aggressive manner to the pressure encountered.

6) *Task Comprehension*

The mentally impaired will often have difficulty understanding verbal directions or instructions. This is often due to the loss of sequential thought - difficulty keeping thoughts in order. This limitation severely restricts basic problem solving. When any task requires more than one step, this person becomes easily confused.

When attempting the task, he may complete the first step and then move onto the second. While performing the second step he will forget the third, and also that he completed the first. If he is not supported through each step, he will become confused by what is required and distressed by the inability to achieve what is desired.

This loss of problem solving ability and difficulty with task comprehension is demonstrated when some mentally impaired are asked to go to the dining room for a meal. The person must first decide which door to take out of the room. When she decides on a door and proceeds through it, she will often stop in her tracks. Her response is not only because she cannot remember where she is going (recent memory loss), but also because she cannot remember where she has come from (loss of sequential thought). She is forced to re-analyze after each location change, and can easily become frustrated by the constant pressure.

This loss of problem solving and sequential thought is often encountered with certain wanderers required to walk a linear path (up and down a straight hallway). When this person reaches a secured door at the end of the hall, he will stop, try the handle and then rock back and forth, standing in that position until someone redirects him. This scenario demonstrates the problem - he wants to go forward, he can't go forward, he cannot remember where he was going, he cannot remember where he was coming from, he cannot figure out how to turn around, and so on. Unless he is assisted with his dilemma, he could become very agitated.

There is an interesting aside to this problem. On a unit housing many mentally impaired clients, this person often has a "buddy wanderer." This is another mentally impaired client who walks with her "friend." When that person is stuck at the door, she grabs him by the arm and re-directs him down the hall. This will often go on all day long. Talk about a support system.

7) *Language*

There are three parts to language changes encountered by some mentally impaired:

- word replacement
- secondary language loss
- language mix

In word replacement, a mentally impaired client develops her own language. As vocabulary is lost, some mentally impaired will find replacement words to communicate what they want - i.e. rag for face cloth, scoop for spoon, cousin for daughter. If the caregiver does not know what she is communicating when using the replacement word, it will create considerable distress.

Secondary language loss results in the person losing a second language and reverting to his primary language. This can occur with an individual who was French speaking, and at the age of forty-five learned English as a second language. Now that he is mentally impaired, he reverts back to speaking French only.

Unfortunately, if those around him (especially family members) are not aware of these dynamics, they may inadvertently pressure him to speak a language that he no longer knows - "My dad can speak English. He has for the past forty years." Unfortunately he has lost English and requires a translator as though he had never learned the second language.

Where some mentally impaired clients will lose their second language completely, others can experience an even more confusing situation called language mix. This can take many forms. Some mentally impaired will be able to understand the secondary language, but only respond in their primary language. Still others will only understand their primary language, but will speak in their secondary language.

A third dynamic of language mix is melding the two languages together. When a person can speak more than one language, then every object, every thought has two distinct words, one from each language. When a person fluent in both English and French wants to talk about a tree, the English word "tree" and the French word "l'arbre" would both come to mind at the same time. This can result in the individual melding the two words together to create a unique type of "gibberish." It may sound like French, but ask a French speaking person to translate and the response will usually be - "That is not French. I do not know what she is saying."

It is sometimes possible to find a consistent sound pattern to this word combination. For example when talking about a tree, the same sound combination seems to replace that word. When the phonetic characteristics of that word combination is discovered, they can be communicated to others by use of a language board (discussed in chapter six).

What is significant about language change is that the client appears to know what he wants to say, but cannot express it in a language that may be familiar to those around him. When those around do not respond appropriately, he can become highly distressed.

8) *Perform*

This is the individual who possesses the cognitive ability to perform a task, but has lost the physical ability to complete it due to progressive apraxia. For example, a mentally impaired client may know how to button his shirt, and what a buttoned shirt looks like, but he cannot seem to make his "fingers work" in order to get the buttons in the hole. His loss of coordination and muscle control prevents him from manually completing the task. If a caregiver is not aware of his limitation, she may inadvertently misinterpret his ability, saying - "I find if you leave him alone with his shirt long enough, he will button it up." There is no question that he may button it, but the distress created in order to complete that task may represent the start of the aggressive cycle.

9) *Environment*

Environmental distressers not only involve noise level as discussed earlier, but any other extreme as well. These can include:

too hot   - wanting the person to take a warm bath when it is stifling outside.

too cold - required to get undressed when the room is too cold.

too dark - cannot make out objects or individuals.

too light - difficult to adjust to the glare creating perceptual problems.

If these issues are not controlled, the mentally impaired can only communicate their inability to cope through their behavioral response.

10) *Disease Process*

The biological cause of aggressive behavior described in chapter two as Volatile Affect is always a possibility. This represented damage to cells in the area of the brain that controls emotional expression. These cells have the ability of "firing" off, stimulating that area and creating a violent response. Unlike circumstantial episodes, this behavior does not seem to have a pattern (discussed in the next chapter).

11) *Values*

This is based on personal values of what is right and decent. It can be encountered when male staff are required to care for a female client. Even though the male staff member may have no difficulty performing the necessary personal care, the client cannot remember where she is and who he is. Therefore, she cannot understand why this male is removing her clothes. Yet she does not resist a female staff performing the same task. The same can occur when female staff are caring for a male client.

Of course with the mentally impaired there is always the exception. There are occasions when female staff are more effective with some male clients than male staff, and male staff are more effective with some female clients than female staff.

Similar dynamics occur for those staff who look young. It is not uncommon for young looking staff to have a mentally impaired older client say - "It's OK *little girl*. I don't need your help." The mentally impaired read the cues as they interpret them They do not see an adult in the features of this staff member, but only a young person. She cannot have a little girl undress her or see her naked, therefore she will probably fight that staff member's attempts to undress, bath or toilet her.

12) *Race*

Some visible minority staff can encounter considerable difficulty while working with certain mentally impaired clients. Asking family, "Is your mother racist?" will get an interesting response. Unless the parent openly professed her racial intolerance, they would probably respond, "My mother was never racist. I never *heard* her say . . ." The key of course is that family "never heard mother say." In actual fact mother may have been racially intolerant when she was cognitively well. However, she knew then that it was not proper to express those ideas and kept many of them to herself. Now that she is mentally impaired she has lost that controlling ability and those hidden beliefs come flying out with every opportunity.

Minority staff cannot personalize these responses. The motivating factor for this person's actions and comments is not the staff member, but the effects of the disease process. It is no different than other staff encountering swearing, degrading or insulting remarks (or having a vase thrown at them). It is simply the person responding to what they encounter, without the controlling ability they once had when they were well.

13) *Past Experience*

This often involves a past history of physical or sexual abuse. An example would be the female client who is fearful of any male caregiver or even male clients, believing that she will be hurt again.

Distress is encountered by any past experiences that have associated with them negative emotions. An excellent example was a Jewish lady who had been in a concentration camp during the war. Now that she was mentally impaired, living on a special unit in a long term care facility, she believed that she was back in that concentration camp. Her assessment was not based on the care, but on her interpretation of the cueing - people were stealing her clothes (to take them to the laundry), she was locked up (security device on the door to prevent elopement behavior), they wouldn't let her out, etc.

14) *Fear of The Unknown*

The fear of the unknown is a common experience for the mentally impaired. They will often resist any object or task that is not familiar. Some of the modern tubs, lifts, chairs, and equipment of today are completely foreign to our older clientele, let alone the mentally impaired. When there is no past memory, one cannot relate to what is occurring in the present.

It is always fascinating to watch staff attempt to place an eighty-seven year old mentally impaired client into a whirlpool tub when he has never seen one before. Even though he may use that tub weekly, his recent memory loss does not allow him to recall the past encounters. If it is not part of "old memory," the person is unable to become familiar with it. The result is an aggressive response with each bath.

Let us personalize this experience to clearly understand the dynamics.

What would be your response if the following occurred to you all within ten minutes?

You are taken into a very bright, sterile room	*. . . you are just getting used to that when you . . .*
see strange equipment and devices	*. . . you are just getting used to that when you . . .*
an unknown person removes your clothes	*. . . you are just getting used to that when you . . .*
are made to sit on a hard, cold chair	*. . . you are just getting used to that when you . . .*
are confined with a security belt	*. . . you are just getting used to that when you . . .*
realize the chair is being lifted into the air	*. . . you are just getting used to that when you . . .*
feel the chair being pushed sideways	*. . . you are just getting used to that when you . . .*
experience the chair being lowered into a box	*. . . you are just getting used to that when you . . .*

realize your feet touch water	*. . . you are just getting used to that when you . . .*
find yourself surrounded by walls	*. . . you are just getting used to that when you . . .*
hear a motor start up	*. . . you are just getting used to that when you . . .*
see the water swirl around	*. . . you are just getting used to that when you . . .*
find it all occurs again in reverse.	

When something is "unknown," a mentally impaired client feels further out of control, anxiety is peaked to a panic level and he will become aggressive.

15) *Being Hurt*

This is often encountered by staff who are small in stature.

Imagine:

> A six foot four, two hundred and forty pound mentally impaired client
> Who has difficulty with balance/
> Being lifted out of a chair
> By a five foot two, one hundred pound caregiver/

Undoubtedly a professional caregiver will have learned the body mechanics to safely maneuver a client of this size. Unfortunately, the client does not know who she is or what she is able to do. A person requires memory retention and analytical ability in order to develop trust with someone.

Simply knowing that a caregiver is a nurse creates for the cognitively well a great deal of comfort or trust. The expectation is that she has had special training to do her job. Likewise, if one can remember that when the caregiver performed the task the last four times, it was done with ease and safety, then the fifth time will present little concern.

The problem confronting a mentally impaired client is that he cannot remember the past four times and cannot remember that she is a skilled caregiver. All he knows is that this "little person" is trying to lift him out of the chair. He is fearful that she will drop him and that will result in his fighting her to leave him alone. On the other hand, the results are different when a staff member with a larger physical stature lifts him from the chair. He does not know that person either, but he feels more comfortable and secure in that person's arms, resulting in his being more cooperative.

16) *Bombarding*

Bombarding occurs when the mentally impaired encounter too much stimuli at one time - either too many instructions, too much noise or too many tasks to complete. Of course with some mentally impaired, bombarding can occur with what we can consider a simple task. Bathing, dressing, eating, or sitting with a small group of people can require the mentally impaired to focus on too much at one time. This will intensify the feeling of being out of control and could result in an aggressive response.

17) *Medication*

We discussed in detail in chapter three how the medication given to stop aggressive behavior can intensify it. The rebound effect experienced with medication use can accelerate the Aggressive Cycle.

18) *Personality Conflict*

Some mentally impaired will relate present events and people to past experiences. If that past experience was negative, then the present encounter will have the same emotions associated with them and create a defensive reaction. Likewise, positive events or relationships of the past can create negative consequences. When a mentally impaired client sees someone she believe she knows or something that she believes she owns, she can become quite agitated when contradicted.

19) *Sensory Loss*

Visual or hearing loss for the mentally impaired are obvious situations that can increase their vulnerability to stimuli and contribute to aggressive outbursts if not adequately adapted. They are not the only situations that must be considered with the mentally impaired. Perceptual difficulties are more common place and in some instances overlooked. A black stripe on the floor is highly confusing (if the stimulus is not intense enough, it will be missed or misinterpreted). It can appear as hole or a step, resulting in the mentally impaired trying to step over it or avoid it.

Likewise a common hearing loss of aging called presbycusis can decrease the ability of the mentally impaired to certain stimuli. A person with presbycusis is able to hear low tones but not high tones. This may mean that the instructions given by male staff may be better understood than those from female staff. Unable to understand the directions by female staff confuses some mentally impaired clients and may result in their becoming aggressive.

20) *Pressure*

Time pressure is probably the most common problem experienced by the mentally impaired. We never seem to have the amount of time for the individual to complete a task, given the amount of time that person requires to complete it.

There is also the potential problem when expectations of performance are too high or too low. When the symptoms are not visible, we are either asking the person to function at a level above her ability or below her ability. The potential for pressure can be a chronic experience for many mentally impaired and cause significant agitation.

21) *Mimicking*

This was presented in both chapter one and two. It refers to the person who is influenced by intense stimuli. Once that stimuli is encountered, this individual will mimic that behavior. If one person is loud, verbal or swearing, this individual will copy that behavior.

22) *Privacy*

This is caused by the inability to know where a person is and that the people around are caregivers. Some mentally impaired are extremely disturbed when someone they do not know is in the room while they are toileting, dressing, bathing, etc.

23) *Sundown Syndrome*

There are two parts to the Sundown Syndrome. One involves energy level. Imagine doing a mentally taxing task for twelve hours without a break. By the twelfth hour, patience and abilities are worn thin. The same is true with the mentally impaired. They are required to concentrate and analyze every noise, face and stimuli every waking minute. By the end of the day, their abilities and tolerance will decrease dramatically.

The cause for increased confusion at night is lighting. When lighting is poor every object has attached to it a shadow. Shadows are obscure stimuli. A room looks one way during the day, and another way in the evening due to the distortion created by the shadows. This perceptual change means that for some mentally impaired clients the room or environment will lose its familiarity as the day advances. Once familiarity is gone, confusion and anxiety may increase, leading to increased agitation.

24) *Lifestyle*

Many people take baths in the morning to wake them up. Others take baths in the evening to help them fall asleep. Give me a bath in the morning when I am eighty-two years old and I will go to bed. If I cannot go to bed, I will sleep in the chair for the next two hours. Put me to bed without the bath and I will be awake for a considerable time afterwards. You cannot change a person's life pattern just because he is in another setting. Doing so can only create unnecessary agitation.

25) *Old Behavior*

The response of some mentally impaired to stress may be no different now than earlier in their lives.

> ⇒ If a person was angered easily in a stressful situation when he was well, the same may occur when he is mentally impaired.
>
> ⇒ If in the past a male client would always use four letter words when angered unless there were women around, he may no longer have that control and uses them regardless of who is around.
>
> ⇒ If a mentally impaired client was always intimidating or always talked in rough and loud voice, that will only increase now when he is distressed.

As we will discover, uncovering past history, personal experiences and personality qualities are key to successfully understanding the mentally impaired.

26) *Physical Discomfort*

The inability to express or analyze what one is feeling makes it hard to communicate verbally when experiencing physical discomfort from hemorrhoids, flu, arthritis, etc. Being asked to perform something else during that discomfort only adds further demands on the individual and will result in an aggressive response.

27) *Control*

It is common for the mentally impaired at some point in their disease to think that they are not sick. Therefore, they feel healthy and in control. This results in their responding to situations and people now based on how they would have responded in the past. This past orientation has a significant influence on behavior.

If a person has nurtured people all through her life, it is possible that she will attempt to continue nurturing people around her now. If she does not believe that she is ill or a resident in long term care facility, then it is easy to see how she can believe that she is there as a volunteer or even a staff member. In fact, it is common to have some mentally impaired clients help staff perform care with others. However, when those same staff turn to this client to take her to the bathroom, she will undoubtedly respond, "No dear that's OK. You help these old people. I don't need your help." The person's belief that she is in control of the situation is confused by the persistence of the staff member to toilet her. Undoubtedly, that can eventually lead to an aggressive response.

28) *Busy*

To others, a mentally impaired client sitting in a chair may not seem to be doing anything. In actual fact, in that person's own mind he is "busy." Whatever recurring past event is being recalled, it is always present. For example, if in a client's mind he believes that he is still on the farm caring for the cows, then he can behave as though it is happening now.

When a caregiver attempts to take that person to the bathroom, he may experience considerable resistance. The reason is simple - he is not done with whatever he believes has to be done at that time, and will not let her lead him away. The more the caregiver persists, the more agitated the client will be with the apparent contradiction.

29) *Bored/Energy Build Up*

An individual who does little each day to expend energy, must find some outlet for it to be expressed. When involved in any task, this individual is often "wound up like a tight spring," and any attempts to control that energy and focus it on a specific task may result in an aggressive response.

30) *Progressive Agitation*

An aggressive episode may be due to things happening to a mentally impaired client that are unknown to the caregiver. For example, if a wandering client pushes the chair of another mentally impaired client each time she walks past, then the agitation level of the one in the chair is continually building. When a staff member approaches the client in the chair, that person may explode into a violent episode without any warning. This client's agitation has progressed over time without anyone being aware of the causative factor.

31) *Confined*

The impact of being confined was demonstrated in chapter two by the client restrained in a chair. It can be seen in more subtle ways as well when the person is blocked from where he wants to go -

- confined to a toilet or commode chair.
- someone blocking a doorway or the hallway.
- not being allowed to go where wants to go.
- teasers (half doors or windows in doors) where he can see the activities of others, but cannot get there.

In each of these cases, his inability to access what he desires will confuse him further and increase the risk of an aggressive response.

32) *False Cueing*

One of my favorite questions asked of staff of a long term care facility is:

"If I were mentally impaired, why is it OK to go to the bathroom in the chair by my bed, but not OK to go to the bathroom in the chair in the lounge?"

Staff are the ones who know that the chair by my bed is a commode chair. The mentally impaired are being asked to respond to contradictory stimuli, and become highly confused as a result.

False cueing implies that a person needs to know where he is before he can understand what is asked of him and what is going on around him. There are many examples of false cueing in a long term care facility.

⇒   I do not wash in my bed (given a basin of water at the bedside).

⇒   I don't go to the bathroom in my bed (urinal or bed pan).

⇒   I am not allowed to go out the door (off the unit), but am allowed to go out the door (secured court yard).

If each of these are not addressed, the mentally impaired can only respond in an aggressive manner.

This lengthy list of causes demonstrates the complexity of this client and his behavior. Unless effective functional assessment tools are employed to define which one or combination of these is specific to the client at hand, then the caregiver is left to guess what is needed to decrease the individual's distress. If the specific causative factor is not addressed, then the potential for a violent episode by some mentally impaired clients is a reality. More importantly, for those mentally impaired who do not respond in a violent manner, the probability of their experiencing significant undue distress for the remainder of their life is high.

SUMMARY

Imagine: A critical care unit in a hospital that has

$\Rightarrow$ no specialized equipment to deal with the serious trauma victims that are housed there.

$\Rightarrow$ staff working on that unit who have had no training in critical care.

Staff will successfully handle situations that their basic training and experience has taught them. Invariably, on a unit with critically ill patients, something more complex and challenging will occur that places the patient's survival in question. Unfortunately, without the necessary tools and skills, the caregivers will be unable to assess the seriousness of a patient's situation until it is severe enough to be obvious to them. By then they may be too late to intervene with anything that may reverse what has occurred. The outcome would definitely place the well being of this patient in jeopardy.

Imagine: A mentally impaired client who is placed in a setting

$\Rightarrow$ geared for the cognitively well.

$\Rightarrow$ with staff who are primarily trained to care for the physically disabled.

$\Rightarrow$ lacking the tools to uncover their needs, the skills to problem solve and the supports to adapt to the individually of the client.

This scenario presents as many difficulties as any critical care unit lacking the same resources. Unfortunately for the mentally impaired, the outcome may not be dramatic enough to initiate the necessary changes, but it would definitely place the well being of this client at risk.

Working with the mentally impaired is a distinct specialty in itself. The skills, tools, philosophy, expectations and approach are not duplicated in any other setting. To achieve a client centered setting with a quality care focus requires specific assessment tools and programming options. It requires the skills of *investigative caregivers*.

Now that the need and response of the mentally impaired has been explained, it is time to define how an *investigative caregiver* does the job effectively.

Chapter Five

ASSESSMENT

The material presented to this point demonstrates the complexity of working with the mentally impaired. It reinforces the basic concept that caring for this clientele does not simply involve following a cookbook or formula type of care. The care strategies employed are totally based on the individual's symptoms and vulnerability. Effective programming must provide a range of care options. The challenge in working with this clientele is to determine what applies to which client at what time. The only way to effectively unravel what is happening and what is needed is to have in place the appropriate investigative tools or specific functional assessment mechanisms.

In *Supportive Therapy*, the goals involved in functional assessment with the mentally impaired elderly are:

1) To identify the individual's strengths and limitations to determine the direction of care.
2) To identify the circumstantial factors that require intervention.

The first goal targets the biological changes created by the disease process. Its focus is to maintain the remaining strengths and compensate for the limitations created by the biological damage that has occurred.

The second goal targets the secondary factors. It focuses on identifying the individual's vulnerability and eliminating the factors that can change behavior and functioning ability. The objectives of functional assessment are quite straightforward. They are to define:

⇒ *what the person can do.*
⇒ *what the person is unable to do.*
⇒ *what distresses the individual further.*

Many of the functional assessment tools defined in this text and the Tactics of Supportive Therapy (Book One) were developed specifically for the technique of *Supportive Therapy*. Likewise, there are an impressive number of alternate assessment tools being utilized within the industry today. All are effective, but not every assessment tool works for every mentally impaired client, or is every assessment tool workable for every caregiver.

Assessing the mentally impaired can be compared to having a set of tools to do a number of different tasks around the home. If you have only one wrench and one screw driver, you will be very limited in what you can perform. There is never a task that has the same size nut or the same type of screw. You need a variety of wrenches and screw drivers to be able to complete the multitude of tasks that can confront you. Likewise, where one handy-person will find it more comfortable to use a short handled screwdriver, another will profess that a long handled one provides more torque, and still another will ascribe to using an electric screw driver only. It really doesn't matter which is used as long as one gets the job done as effectively as the other.

The same is true with assessment. There is no one assessment tool that is better than another in many cases. As long as the outcome (the needed information to be uncovered) is obtained, then the process of how it was obtained is not as significant.

It is expected that where one caregiver is comfortable with one assessment tool, another caregiver may find an alternate easier to use. The freedom for this type of individuality is the key to success. However:

An organization needs to have a defined standardization of tools to ensure consistency in the information obtained.

The following tools may be used as described, incorporated with those already in use in your organization, adapted to fit your organization, or you may find that what you now use accomplishes the same outcome.

A caution! The challenge of writing about assessment tools (as well as programming options) is that there is limited space to discuss all situations where these might be employed. Unfortunately, some believe that when they read something they must do it exactly as defined in every situation. With this clientele that is not practical. It is impossible to define every situation that each individual mentally impaired client might create or demonstrate. Therefore it is impossible to be thorough enough to answer all of the concerns. Flexibility and creativity to adjust the tools at hand is one of the many skills of the investigative caregiver. As long as you are client centered, the client will tell you when what you are doing is not appropriate or acceptable.

OVERVIEW OF ASSESSMENT STRATEGIES

This text is not intended to duplicate the material from my other texts unless it deals specifically with aggressive behavior. What is provided in the upcoming pages is an overview of many of the Supportive Therapy Assessment Strategies. The following code identifies the text in which the material is located.

ST - *The Tactics of Supportive Therapy*
GSE - *Getting Staff Excited*
M - *Mother I'm Doing The Best I Can*
PAA - *described in the following chapters*

Organizational Assessment

Staff Needs Assessment (GSE)
A detailed questionnaire assessing the supports provided to staff that will empower them to perform their job effectively and efficiently.

Evaluating The Care Process for
The Mentally Impaired Elderly (ST)
A comprehensive questionnaire that allows an organization to measure it's thoroughness in programming and define the strengths and limitations as determined by staff and managers.

Precursors To Aggressive Behavior (PAA)

> A measuring tool that defines the working environment
> and how it may contribute to the aggressive response of
> the mentally impaired.

Care Assessment

Client Profile (PAA)

> A detailed questionnaire defining the base line data
> required to effectively work with the individual
> clientele.

Patterning (ST/PAA)

> A behavioral assessment tool to uncover the time and
> cause of specific behaviors.

Care Analysis (ST/PAA)

> A team assessment tool utilized during the care
> conference.

24 Hour Profile (ST)

> An assessment of individual functioning ability and
> effective strategies already employed to support the
> individual.

Medical (ST)

> The components of a basic medical assessment to ensure
> that the individual is experiencing an irreversible
> dementia and also define possible secondary factors
> (disease, drugs).

Family

Family Questionnaire (ST/M)

> These are two separate questionnaires. One attempts to
> uncover from family what they know about the client
> since the person has become impaired. The other

attempts to uncover for family what issues must be resolved in order for family to cope with this ordeal.

Thought Transition

Diversional Tactics (PAA)
Attempting to uncover what will illicit negative emotions and what thought process will capture positive emotions.

Progressive Functioning (PAA)
This tool is used to determine the change in functioning ability from first contact.

Interview (ST)

Attention Span
Defining the length of time the client can concentrate on a specific task.

Emotional State
Defining the recurrent emotional state that will arise with any situation.

Language Pattern
Defines the word replacement, language mix and language loss that may be experienced.

Thought Process
Determines the logic process retained by this person in discussions.

Reminiscing Ability
Uncovers what can be discussed that will change thought process and emotional state.

Perceptual Assessment (ST)

> Questions defining the client's orientation and as a
> result the subsequent behavioral response to specific
> stimuli.

Activities of Daily Living

Comprehension Board (PAA)
> This tool is used to define verbal, task and performance
> comprehension.

Task Assessment (ST)
> This assessment process is intended to discover
> response to activities of daily living requirements.

Environmental Assessment (ST)

> Identifies the individual's ability to utilize environmental cueing
> techniques including: Color
>   Word Comprehension
>   Object Identification
>   Clock and Event Board Assessment

Medication

Dosage & Dispensing Pattern (PAA)
> Used to define specific patterns of behavior in order to
> discover causative factors and alternate intervention
> strategies.

Three Month Review (ST)
> Implemented to challenge medication usage, to
> determine whether the drug can be decreased or
> discontinued.

Trial Period Without (ST)
>Employed to decrease medication use to personal tolerance level or discontinue completely when alternate strategies are employed.

Past Profile

Historical Profile (ST/PAA)
>Tools employed to define and monitor specifics about the client's background and personality qualities that may explain certain behavioral characteristics.

Aggressive Episodes (PAA)
>An analysis process of aggressive/violent episodes to uncover possible causative factors.

Organizational assessment tools will be discussed in chapter eight on staffing. The following assessment tools are detailed in The Tactics of Supportive Therapy and not discussed in this text: medical, task, family, 24 hour profile and environmental assessment. The remainder will be outlined in this chapter (with reference to Book One): medication, care assessment, interview, historical profile and aggressive pattern.

UNCOVERING SECRETS

In reality, the basic assessment tool employed in working with the mentally impaired is trial and error. Often there is no way to know the abilities, limitations or vulnerabilities of an individual until something that distresses this person is encountered. Therefore the primary source to determine what works and what doesn't are those caregivers who have had the most contact with the individual (whether professional caregivers or family members). Based on their experiences, they can often define what this person can and cannot do, and what distresses this individual. Unfortunately there may be "secrets" in many care settings.

The term secrets implies that individuals within the care team or family members may have information about the client that is not known by others involved in this person's care. Unfortunately in some settings that information is not readily available. The reasons secrets exist are many:

⇒ the information is subtle and not conscious to the primary caregiver(s).
⇒ the opportunity may not be there to share it.
⇒ the person may not think that it is important.
⇒ it may be believed that it is already known by others.
⇒ the caregiver may have a skill(s) that is unique compared to what others are employing.
⇒ the caregiver may not be confident in his/her ability to express it to other professionals.
⇒ there may not be a formal tool in place to uncover it.

Any investigation into a client's behavior must first uncover in detail what those caregivers already know. Many of the tools presented in the following pages "tap the brain" of existing caregivers. It is often the case that somebody has the key that will unlock the mystery behind this client's behaviors. If that information can be shared with everyone, then all will increase their success with that individual.

It is only when all of the secrets or existing information is exposed, that there is a need to impose any alternate assessment tools to reveal what no one has resolved as yet. It is easy to demonstrate the importance of uncovering secrets when assessing for something called Pre-emptive Cueing.

PRE-EMPTIVE CUEING

There is often no need to tell someone when a person is aggressive. Knowing when a person has become aggressive is often quite obvious. The question that must be asked of primary caregivers is "How can you tell when the person will become aggressive, before he becomes aggressive?"

The majority of mentally impaired clients often have some mannerism, expression or behavior that indicates that they are distressed. This information defines what is called the Pre-emptive Cueing. Staff or family who know this individual have often experienced that pre-warning cue. The cueing can be a variety of unique signals, such as restlessness, picking at clothing, mumbling, pacing, tapping, specific words expressed, etc. The assessment questions that must be asked of those who care for this individual are:

> *How do you know when the person is becoming*
> *distressed?*
> *What do you do when you encounter it?*

You will often hear a caregiver say, "You just look for the face." This demonstrates how subtle the cueing can be. The caregiver has identified the non-verbal behavior that communicates when the client is distressed. She knows that if she does not react to that cueing appropriately, then the client will soon become aggressive.

It is important for the caregiver to describe "the face" and then record that description on the client's chart or care plan. Once the pre-emptive cueing is formally identified, those who have less contact or have not uncovered that information will be able to prevent aggressive outbursts from occurring.

In some instances it may be difficult for the caregiver to describe what is encountered. In that case, it is important that each time "the face" or cueing is seen, then it is shown to others involved in this person's care. This requires drawing another caregiver over at the time and stating "That is the face!"

PATTERNING

This is probably one of the most valuable assessment tools that can be employed in understanding the needs of the mentally impaired. The mentally impaired seem to always demonstrate a pattern to their behavior (excluding volatile affect). The purpose of this assessment tool is to define that pattern in order to identify the intervention strategy needed to decrease or eliminate the distresser. There are two components to patterning - the time pattern and the event pattern.

Patterning can be used to investigate any behavior - aggression, sexually expressive behavior, rummaging, etc. To define the time pattern, caregivers are asked to monitor the behavior over a set period of time. The assessment period usually ranges from one to three weeks, depending on the type, incidence and circumstances of the behavior. During that defined period, the caregiver is to record the time the behavior occurs and the duration of the episode.

To define the event pattern, the caregiver is required to describe what is going on around and to the person at that time. They are not to evaluate the situation, but only describe the circumstances the individual client is experiencing. Once that information is recorded over the set period, it is then examined to see if it discloses a time and/or event pattern.

By the way, staff who know this client will often have assessed this pattern intuitively on their own. It is common to hear caregivers comment:

"He always becomes agitated in the afternoon."
"She always wanders more after lunch."
"He fidgets more in the evening"

They have informally defined the time pattern. When it is completed formally by the entire care team, it provides valuable information on the care strategies required to define programming needs.

Let us take an example to demonstrate the value of patterning. Imagine that the pre-emptive cueing is swearing. Certain caregivers know that when the client is swearing, it indicates that she will soon become physically aggressive if supports are not implemented.

Each time swearing is encountered, caregivers are asked to identify the time it occurs and describe what is going on around or to that person at that time. When the caregivers complete their assessment and compare the results they discover that the individual demonstrates this behavior every afternoon around 1400 hours. Records of the behavior indicate that the times vary from 1330 to 1430 hours. When they describe what is going on around or to this person, it uncovers the potential causative factor. The client normally sits in the lounge every afternoon after lunch. Every day at around 1330 hours there is a recreational activity scheduled in the lounge. This client begins swearing around 1400 hours. It is obvious that she cannot tolerate the stimuli created by the activity. The solution is to remove her from the lounge at 1320 hours or move the activities out of the lounge.

Often the solution is that simple. Once the individual's behavior pattern is uncovered, it usually leads to the potential causative factor creating it. Once known, the care option employed to resolve that factor is usually quite easy to define. This tool is highly valuable to provide direction to the care team.

Unfortunately, the event pattern is the most difficult to define. There may not always be an obvious connection between the descriptions each time the behavior is encountered. However, the time pattern is nearly always uncovered.

Let's go back to our example of the person swearing every day around two o'clock. Although the descriptions of what is going on around or to the person at or before that time do not uncover the causative factor, knowing the time pattern is valuable. It defines a programming need. This client requires an activity or diversion to redirect her energy in a more productive and acceptable manner, to change her thought process, and to be removed from the stresser (even though we may know what it is). Each of these will be discussed in the next chapter on programming.

The information for patterning can come from three sources:

⇒ *Formal Assessment*
⇒ *Consistent Staff*
⇒ *PRN Medication*

1) Formal Assessment Mechanism - Utilizing patterning as a formal assessment tool provides the most valuable and accurate information.

2) Consistent Staff - if detailed record keeping of the behavior in question is not in place, then interviewing those who work consistently with this client will often define the time pattern. Unfortunately, the opportunity to contact every caregiver in a health care setting that may have information on this client is time consuming. Likewise, to expect those caregivers to recall specifically what was going on around and to the client during each of those times is unlikely. Therefore, the ability to discover the event pattern is even more difficult.

3) PRN Medication - if staff are not consistent, and no one has that detailed knowledge of the individual, then the third way is by examining the administration of PRN medication.

In one case the time pattern was defined after examining the medication record for the previous three months. It was discovered that the PRN sedation was administrated every day between 1500 and 1630 hours and every morning between 0300 and 0500 hours. When the client profile (discussed later in this chapter) was completed and this client's day was mapped, it became obvious what was occurring.

The client in question was low functioning and had a poor attention span. Other than activities of daily living (washing, dressing and eating), there was minimal programming scheduled throughout the day. She would get up from bed at 0630 hours. Between 0630 and 0800 hours, morning care was completed and breakfast was eaten. The remainder of the day she would sit in the lounge. With nothing to focus on or occupy time, she would simply doze off in the chair. At 1000 hours, staff would wake for her morning snack and take her to the washroom. Back in the chair again, she would nap for another half hour or so. She would then have lunch, return to the lounge again and doze off for a period.

As the day progressed, she would become increasingly restless (pre-emptive cueing). By late afternoon, she was aggressive, fighting all procedures and striking out at anyone near her. Hence the need for sedation at that time (1500 to 1630 hours). After the sedation she would become drowsy and sleep until supper. After supper, she would return to the lounge and doze in the chair again for up to an hour.

This client was normally in bed by 2000 hours. Most mornings she would awaken between 0100 and 0300 hours, raring to go. If staff tried to settle her back to bed, she would become loud and aggressive. She would then receive the PRN sedation. When the pattern of medication dispensing was uncovered, programming was then implemented to occupy the client's time and exhaust her energy throughout the day. That resulted in a dramatic decrease in the use of PRN medication, as well as a decrease in her aggressive outbursts.

Using the PRN ordering pattern and/or interviewing consistent staff as an assessment tool is valuable. Unfortunately they require piecing information after the fact, which is very time consuming and does not usually provide enough information to uncover the event pattern. Formally utilizing the technique of Patterning is the most accurate and thorough. It substantiates the concept that the mentally impaired will always communicate by their behavior, and it ensures that we don't miss what they are trying to tell us.

PROCESS OF CARE ANALYSIS

Care analysis is a problem identification mechanism utilized during the care conference. It allows all members of the care team to brainstorm what may be causing a client's behavior or change in functioning. A summary of the procedure is as follows:

⇒ At a the care conference, a flip chart is placed in front of the care team and a staff member is asked to become the recorder.

⇒ The recorder's job is to first write on the flip chart a concern or behavior (called a care issue) staff are having difficulty with regarding a specific client (i.e. wandering, aggression, hoarding, etc.).

⇒ All staff are then asked to give all of the possible reasons why any client who is mentally impaired may perform in that manner.

⇒ Once all of the reasons are identified, staff are asked which causative factor on the list they believe applies to this client.

⇒ This becomes the care diagnosis on the resident/client care plan.

Let us take aggression as an example of the care analysis process at work. During a care conference, the care team identifies that a client becomes aggressive during meal times. This is considered the care issue and placed on the top of the flip chart.

Staff are then asked to identify all of the possible reasons why any mentally impaired client may respond in this manner. We have spent the time to detail the 32 causes of aggressive behavior (discussed in the previous chapter). Normally that information is not readily available to staff on all care issues encountered. Therefore they would be required to develop the list on their own.

Each potential cause is listed below the care issue on the flip chart. When their brainstorming is complete, the flip chart sheet would have the following information:

Aggressive During Meal Times

Depression	Medication
Time	Personality Conflict
Timing	Sensory Loss
Approach	Pressure
Word Comprehension	Mimicking
Task Comprehension	Privacy
Language	Sundown Syndrome
Perform	Lifestyle
Environment	Old Behavior
Disease Process	Physical Discomfort
Values	Control
Race	Busy
Past Experience	Bored/Energy Build-up
Fear of the Unknown	Progressive Agitation
Being Hurt	Confined
Bombarding	False Cueing

Once discussion of the possible causes is completed, the care team is asked "Which of these do you believe applies to this person?" Those caregivers who consistently work with this individual may identify that she cannot handle "bombarding." They have discovered that if she is given too many instructions or things to do at one time, then she will usually become distressed, and at times aggressive. They have aptly identified the care diagnosis for this client's care plan:

Aggressive during meal times
possibly related to bombarding.

Once a possible causative factor is revealed, the intervention strategies are straightforward - give her one thing to do, one instruction at a time, plus remove her from situations that have multiple stimuli. Those are then implemented into the care process for a set period of time before re-evaluating. If there is no change in her aggressive response, then the situation must be reassessed again.

If aggressive behavior during meal times continues, then at another care conference the care team is required to scan the original list of possible causes again. This time they are asked - "What else may contribute to her difficulty with meal time?" Certain staff may indicate that she requires a specific approach. If anyone approaches her from the side without warning, she becomes very distressed. The care diagnosis is now expanded to:

Aggressive during meal time
possibly related to an inappropriate approach

The care team again implements the needed intervention strategies to ensure that the appropriate approach during meal time is taken. If there is no noted change in behavior, then the team must re-assess again. We will discuss in the next chapter on programming the significance of this process in defining behavior.

The Care Analysis Process works on the basis that aggression is a *symptom* of an *underlying problem* (causative factor). Programming for the mentally impaired is based totally on what the individual is encountering. Until the causative factor is uncovered, then there is little direction on programming needs. The technique of care analysis has a number of benefits:

1) **Group Knowledge Sharing** - It formalizes the group's analysis process during the care conference to ensure thorough assessment.

2) **Information Sharing** - Those who know the client the best, can share with others what may be affecting that person specifically.

3) Individualizes the Care Plan - Where one causative factor results in one person reacting in a certain way, another person reacting in the same way will have a different causative factor. This process ensures that programming is specific to the symptoms and vulnerability of the individual client.

4) Teaching Tool - It demonstrates the complexity of the client to all involved. It is not simply a black/white analysis, but a highly complex situation. Participants are taught how to analyze and problem solve what is experienced.

5) Communication Tool - It ensures that all involved have the same information about the client and understand the rationale behind the direction taken.

6) Time Efficiency - It provides a format for the care conference that focuses attention, time and efforts towards a common goal.

This technique can be used with any behavior, with any type of client. It is highly effective in ensuring the individuality and specifics of client care.

CLIENT PROFILE *(Actual form is located in the addendum, page 203)*

It is important when assessing a client to periodically take a snap shot of what is occurring. This summary overview, or client profile, provides a detailed assessment that will often uncover secrets, patterns, relationship of behaviors, response to schedules and events, etc.

A client profile includes the following:

Past History - what do you know about this individual regarding: family, work, accomplishments, likes/dislikes, leisure activities, etc.

Rationale - This is intended to define past memories that may relate to the behaviors encountered today. There are many examples:

Behavior	Past History
Client goes into the rooms of others.	Past minister who frequently visited people in nursing homes.
Stripping flowered wall paper.	Enjoyed gardening.
Fearful of male staff and clients.	Abused sexually at youth.
Concerned about the "baby being hurt."	Cared for a sick child.
Urinating in waste basket.	Farmer with no indoor plumbing.
Always straightening and cleaning.	Meticulous housekeeper.

Personality Characteristics - Identify what you know about this person regarding self image (dress and appearance), how this person dealt with stress in the past, dependency on others, rituals, dominant personality qualities, etc.

Rationale - Intended to define pre-morbid personality traits that are carried over from the past:

Behavior	Past History
Swearing.	Normal vocabulary for individual.
Constantly straightening clothing.	Always meticulous at how she was dressed.
Fearful when alone.	Highly dependent, rarely alone when well.
Will not eat breakfast.	Never has eaten until later in the day.

Present State - What behaviors or symptoms does this person demonstrate? When do they occur? (if known)

Rationale - The first question attempts to identify which behaviors need to be examined and the linkage of a symptom to a behavior (progressive apraxia and aggression when attempting to button his shirt). The second attempts to define any suspected patterns to those behaviors.

Medication History -

1) *Present Drug Regime*
   Drug Ordered/Dosage/ Frequency/Reason Ordered/
   Date Order Began

2) *Past Drug Regime*
   Drug Ordered/Dosage/Frequency/Reason Ordered/
   Date Began/Date Discontinued/Reason Discontinued

   Rationale: Both of these are used to uncover a potential rebound effect as discussed in the previous chapter, where one drug is ordered to deal with a behavior, then increased, and then another added, etc. The information gained in answering this question relates to one of the questions under the following section called *point of change*.

If PRN sedation is being used - Drug Order/Dosage/
   Times Given (over past three months)

   Rationale: As described, mapping the times a PRN sedation is administered is one of the ways to uncover a behavior pattern.

Daily Profile - Outline this individual's normal day, identifying hour by hour activities of daily living, how time is spent, recreational activities, etc. Define what this person does in detail and the individual's response to each event. Add at the bottom anything done weekly or monthly, i.e. bath or certain recreational activities, etc.

Rationale: Examining a daily log of events uncovers patterns, holes in programming that may contribute to behavioral response, contradictions in scheduling to life pattern, etc.

Point of Change - Identify a time in the recent past where this person looked, acted or performed differently than what would be seen today. Describe that person back then, including behavior, abilities, care needs, etc. that would not be seen today.

Rationale: The answer to this question in conjunction with the information on the past and present medication regime identifies a point of change. Investigating what occurred at that point may lead to uncovering a secondary factor.

When is this person's "worse time" of the day? - How will the person respond (behavior, refusal/inability to perform tasks) during that time? What usually occurs around or to the client during and after that time?

Rationale: This is looking for pre-emptive cueing and a pattern of behavior, as well as the response by caregivers during that time.

What is required to settle the individual? - What will be the result? How long before he/she will return to "his/her normal self?"

Rationale: These questions are attempting to uncover information on programming options employed and the response encountered.

Enhancing Functioning Ability - What needs to be told to a "new" caregiver about this client that will allow that person to be successful?

Rationale: Again this attempts to uncover information known by consistent caregivers that has not been communicated within the care plan or chart.

What would you like to see different about this client than what is being done now? - Regarding care, activities, medication, treatment, etc.

> *Rationale:* This question attempts to draw from caregivers their creativity on programming alternatives that have not been employed with this client.

The client profile is first completed by the caregiver who has the most contact with the client in question. It is then reviewed by the care team to add or delete information as required. The information is then examined to draw out any issues that require alternate intervention strategies.

HISTORICAL PROFILE

1) Client Log

It can take up to a year or longer to compile a complete historical profile on a mentally impaired client. The social history and more general facts about this person's background are usually readily available on admission. Unfortunately, in many settings, the client's history is usually filed within the chart and not expanded again. However, the more personal details are more gradual in coming. It is these that are often crucial to understanding the individual's behavior. This information is usually obtained by casual conversations with family members, acquaintances and other caregivers who knew the client in the past.

- In one case staff knew that the client was a minister, but few knew that years ago he was the visiting minister for the facility where he now lived. His need to go in and out of rooms linked well with his past memory.
- In another case, a staff member learned from family that the client was claustrophobic. Once the client was placed on a small stool in the tub, she stopped fighting

bath time. It seemed that the sides of the tub frightened her.

- In another case, the work history of an agitated wanderer was only known as a laborer. It was during an informal conversation with family that it was discovered their father was a sweeper for the past twenty seven years. Once known, he was given a broom and encouraged to sweep the hallway floor. His agitation was eliminated.

In each of these cases the information was known by specific caregivers only, but not know by others until it was disclosed in the Client Profile.

It is always a pleasure to watch another caregiver's response when an unknown piece of information is shared with the care team. It is often stated with a perspicuous expression - "I didn't know about that." It is almost as though a light goes on to explain why the client is behaving in a certain way.

There is no doubt that certain caregivers will achieve a better rapport with family and glean more information than others. That cannot be unintentionally hoarded. In order to keep information current, it is valuable to create a Client Log. This is a blank form with the heading Client Log at the top. This form should be kept at the very front of the client's chart. Staff are then instructed to record anything they discover about this client from any source (other than confidential information).

The more information that can be uncovered the clearer the picture may be about the client's aggressive behavior, and the more accurate the direction on what can be done to resolve it.

2) Past History

There are specific questions that the family must be asked to understand a client's aggressive behavior. It is usually family who are the only ones who can relate what is happening now with what occurred in the past. When the past can be linked, it will often provide direction on necessary intervention strategies. Three of the assessment questions family are asked include:

> ⇒ *Describe your mom/dad to me twenty years ago.*
> ⇒ *How has your mom/dad dealt with stress all through their life?*
> ⇒ *Identify significant events that stand out in your mom/dad's life for you.*

Describe your mother to me 20 years ago. - The response to this question can identify qualities or traits of this individual that may be influencing certain behavioral reactions.

In one organization, staff identified on the Client Profile that the client's worst time of day was first thing in the morning. When her daily log was examined, it indicated that staff would wake this client at 0630 hours, get her washed, dressed and then feed her breakfast all by 0800 hours. When family were asked to describe their mother twenty years ago regarding this routine they responded - "Mother never liked getting up early." The care routine can never effectively change a client's life pattern. When she was allowed to get up later, she had less difficulty handling the demands placed upon her and her aggression was eliminated.

How has your mom/dad dealt with stress throughout life? - This question attempts to define pre-morbid personality qualities. When asked, family may respond that when their dad was stressed "the air around him was blue." Now that he is mentally impaired, he may always be stressed, therefore the air can always be "blue." Once this is uncovered as old behavior, family can provide the care team significant direction of how his behavior can be approached. Knowing that the daughters always joked with their father to snap him out of his "bad mood," becomes a valuable intervention strategy now.

Identify significant events that stand out in your mom/dad's life for you? Memory is selective. We do not remember every minute of every day. Memories generally have strong positive or negative emotions associated with them.

If you have children
Go back into your past/
To the first day
You brought your first child home/
Lift your eyes from the page for a moment to experience
that event/

As you remember that time, you will probably smile. That day for most has associated with it strong emotion, making it is easy to recall. The next question will not be so easy to answer. What happened the seventh, eleventh, or thirty-fifth day? If nothing occurred on those days to stir any emotion, then they will virtually be impossible to remember.

Memory is selective. The strongest memories are events that have associated with them strong emotions, either positive or negative. The assessment question - Identify a time in your mom/dad's past that stands out for you (the family member) - provides significant insight. If it is easily recalled by the offspring, then it probably was quite vivid for the parent. We have now identified possible bench marks of memory loss. Identifying these benchmarks provides two components of programming:

Past events that create negative emotions should be avoided (called taboos).

Past events that create positive emotions can be used (called distracters).

3) Aggressive Profile

Who has less of a problem or no problem?
Who has the most difficulty with this client?

Who has less of a problem or no problem? - identifies who may have the greatest rapport with a specific client. Encountering certain caregivers having a greater rapport with a specific client is common. They are often caregivers who have features that link them with individuals the client knew in the past. Being able to recognize those qualities in that caregiver increases familiarity (which decreases anxiety), or even results in the client believing the caregiver is that person.

In one example, a client would fight all caregivers except one on every aspect of activities of daily living. The caregiver she cooperated with was tall, blonde and blue eyed. Apparently a long time friend of this client during her youth had the same features. The client thought the caregiver was that friend and cooperated fully. A staff member who is perceived this way is valuable in a number of instances. This caregiver can:

⇒ be useful during stressful times by becoming a distracter for the client, able to influence or even change this person's emotional state.

⇒ provide other caregivers specific information and direction on effective programming strategies that can be used with this client.

⇒ complete the more difficult or stressful tasks for this client in order to decrease the distress experienced.

Who has the most difficulty with this client? - This is not intended to ostracize staff who do not perform their jobs well (although it frequently does uncover that). It attempts to identify personality conflicts between a client and a caregiver. As often as some caregivers are perceived as someone positive from their past, other caregivers may be viewed as someone negative from their past. This conflict with certain caregivers can be due to:

• fear of the individual (male caregiver, small stature, looks young, etc.).

• intolerance (race, gender).

• personality conflict (beard, etc.).

When a mentally impaired client associates a caregiver with negative emotions, it will be almost impossible for that person to work effectively with that client. In this case, it is simply the client relating something about that person to a past distressful memory.

THE INTERVIEW

Using the interview as an assessment tool with low functioning mentally impaired clients can be the most challenging. A functional assessment interview is <u>not intended</u> to prove that the person is confused and disoriented, unable to maintain a conversation for any period of time, or has difficulty with analytical thought. With the low functioning mentally impaired, those symptoms are well defined already. Interviewing the mentally impaired has a more unique rationale that may uncover some meaningful and important information.

THE CHALLENGES OF CONDUCTING AN INTERVIEW

It is not uncommon to see some professionals conduct an interview with the mentally impaired client in the same manner as they would interview a cognitively well client. The error in their approach can include any one of the following - they will:

- ⇒ often set a pre-determined length for the interview.
- ⇒ position themselves inappropriate to the client.
- ⇒ lack the necessary base line data.
- ⇒ conduct a series of questions as though it were an interrogation.
- ⇒ ignore the cues from the client.
- ⇒ not establish the necessary rapport.
- ⇒ not know the taboos that should be avoided.

It is not surprising that the results from their interview will often be inaccurate.

One cannot just sit down with a mentally impaired client and begin a conversation. Conducting an interview is often stressful for the client.

It involves intense stimuli. A face-to-face interaction with someone that is not familiar, who is pressuring the individual to perform.

1) Base Line Information

No interview can be conducted with the mentally impaired until the base line information about the client is discovered. It is too easy to increase this individual's anxiety level, which will decrease the person's functioning level and skew the results of the interview. An effective interviewer first interviews the caregivers before interviewing the mentally impaired client. That requires answers to the following questions.

What distresses the individual?

What are the taboos (things not to discuss)?

What are the pre-emptive cues to warn that the individual is distressed?

What are the distracters that can be employed should the person become distressed?

How should the person be approached?

Are their existing communicative limitations beyond mental impairment (i.e. hearing problems)?

What can the person talk about easily?

Who are the family members and where are they living (to provide topics of conversation and determine the accuracy of what the client is describing)?

What is the individual's past history - employment, spouse, where lived (also to provide topics of conversation and determine accuracy)?

Who is the best caregiver to introduce the interviewer to the client?

Does that person need to stay for a period?

Where is the client's most comfortable location?

What is required to establish the greatest rapport?

2) Time Limitation

There can be no pre-determined time limit when interviewing the mentally impaired. The client will define the maximum amount of time he/she can tolerate the interview process. With some mentally impaired, the conversation can last twenty minutes or longer. With others, it could be as short as a couple of minutes and only two questions before the client will want to leave. Making the person sit in the chair for a longer period so that the interview can be completed will not only provide limited information on the client's ability, but will also increase the individual's distress level, leaving the caregiver with a potentially agitated client.

Interviewing the mentally impaired is often something that is conducted over an extended period of time. The interviewer makes periodic contact (until the person's tolerance level is exhausted), then returns later to carry on with the interview.

3) Style

The successful interview ensures that the client does not feel as though she/he is being interrogated. If the mentally impaired feel as though they are being questioned, it will only increase their anxiety, skewing the interview and increasing the potential for an aggressive response. The interview must take on the form of a conversation, sprinkled with specific questions and watching for the pre-emptive cueing that indicates that the person is becoming distressed. Once that distress is encountered, the interviewer must either change the topic or end the interview if necessary.

Establishing rapport or trust with this client is essential before any interview can take place. The location where the interview is conducted must be the one that holds the greatest familiarity for this client. That may mean that some interviews are conducted on the run (walking with a wandering client).

One of the least effective ways to begin an interview is:

not to be introduced to the client by a caregiver.

or

to be introduced by a caregiver who distresses the client.

In the first situation there is no associated familiarity. It is a "cold contact" and anxiety will be increased immediately. In the second case, the interviewer will only encounter the client saying - "You are with her." The immediate link with the caregiver makes it difficult for the interviewer to establish any rapport with the client.

Being introduced to the client by a caregiver or family member who has the greatest rapport will often result in the client being more comfortable with the interviewer. Rapport is virtually "passed on" from the caregiver to the interviewer. With more sensitive clients, it may be necessary to have that caregiver or family member stay during part or all of the interview to comfort the client even further.

BENEFITS OF THE INTERVIEW

Using the interview as a functional assessment tool has many benefits. Some of these have already been addressed:

Attention Span - Defining the length of time the client can
> concentrate on a specific task.

Emotional State - Defining the recurrent emotional state that
> will arise with any situation.

Language Pattern - Defines the word replacement, language
> mix and language loss that may be experienced.

Thought Process - Determines the logic process retained by this
> person in discussions.

Reminiscing Ability - Uncovers what can be discussed that will
> change thought process and emotional state.

These have been discussed in detail in the text The Tactics of Supportive Therapy. There is another benefit to the interview that was presented in the case example in chapter two - the opportunity to assess thought transition.

Assessing thought transition involves determining how long it takes the person's thought process to catch up with the actions of others. This is conducted in the following manner. Four questions are asked within the opening minutes of the interview (intermixed within the conversation to avoid the feeling of being interrogated). These same four questions are repeated again at the five to six minute mark. The questions are as follows:

How old are you?
What year were you born?
Who is in this picture (family portrait)?
What is your spouse's name?

In the case example in chapter two, the client demonstrated well what can occur. When asked these four questions in the first minute or two, he did not answer any of them. When asked at the five minute mark he was able to answer the last three questions (19, 19, 19, 1920; cousin, cousin; Mary).

The difference in functioning between the first few minutes and the five to six minute mark is significant. The interview was conducted as follows:

> The interview was conducted at the end of a two day assessment of the unit. During that two day period, a number of staff were interviewed about this client to establish the base line information. The client profile and 24 hour profile were completed. Repeated contacts were made with this client in a number of settings in order to establish rapport and familiarity (ate meals with him, wandered the hall with him, sat with him in the lounge). The interview was conducted late the second day in the client's room (familiar environment), with the door closed (to decrease stimuli). A caregiver with the greatest rapport was asked to be in the client's room at the beginning of the interview.

Regardless of the preparation, my presence and the demands of the task initially elevated his anxiety level. (When anxiety is increased, mental functioning decreases). During this initial period, he was incapable of concentrating on the task. He was bombarded by the amount of stimuli encountered (a secondary factor) and had difficulty understanding the initial questions.

After the five minute mark he became more comfortable and less threatened by my presence. His anxiety level decreased, his awareness increased and he was able to respond more appropriately. The secondary factor was lessened and he was able to perform at his true functioning level.

The client required a specific amount of time for his thought process to catch up with the activity at hand. That is important for staff to know. If those doing his personal care gave instructions on first contact, then he will not likely respond to their direction. Should they pressure him to follow those instructions, he will invariably become distressed and aggressive. Within the first few moments of contact, he is too easily distracted by what is occurring. However, starting with the least demanding task, then giving instructions after he is accustomed to her presence, may result in his being more cooperative.

This information becomes important for all aspects of care - bathing, meal time, dressing, recreational activities, etc. Giving this gentleman instructions on first contact will result in his not responding. If staff are more gradual in their demands, his comprehension and ability to complete the task will improve.

Thought transition attempts to discover how long it takes a client's thought process to catch up with the actions around him. Once discovered, it is a tremendous asset in determining how programming is presented to the client.

COMPREHENSION BOARD

There are many forms of this type of board. It is often a plywood tray that can be secured to the arms of a chair with Velcro strips. On the tray are pieces of cloth with buttons of varying sizes, a zipper, laces, Velcro strips, hook/eye (from a brassiere), belt, neck tie, etc. This is a simple homemade device that is intended to uncover:

* *word/object association*
* *task comprehension*
* *manual ability*
* *attractors*

This assessment must be completed by the caregiver with the greatest rapport and in an area free from other stimuli. The tray is placed in front of the client. The client is then asked to fasten the buttons by giving the following instructions:

1) *Verbal Direction* - The client is simply told, "Please fasten the buttons." If he fastens the buttons without difficulty then he is moved to the next object.

2) *Verbal Direction, Pointing To The Object* - If he does not move to the buttons on verbal instruction, then he is given the same instructions again with the caregiver pointing to the buttons at the same time. If he responds and fastens the buttons, then he probably no longer understands the word "buttons," but he understands what to do when he sees them. The care team will know that asking him to fasten his buttons is insufficient. Pointing to them, as well as asking him, will result in his performing without further assistance.

3) *Attempts Task, But Unable to Complete* - If on verbal instruction or by pointing, he attempts to fasten the buttons, but is unsuccessful, then he is possibly demonstrating something else. In this case, he may have the cognitive ability to understand the task, but has lost coordination or manual ability to complete it. Therefore, he cannot be pressured to do the task on his own, or he will probably become distressed.

4) *Attractor* - Should the client continually return to the buttons regardless of any other requests to the contrary. He fastens the buttons, unfastens them, fastens them, unfastens them and so on. The buttons may be an attractor. They are an intense stimuli that the individual cannot avoid. Therefore buttons on clothing may have to be replaced with snaps, zipper or Velcro tape to prevent him from exposing himself.

This assessment process is repeated for each of the articles.

RECREATIONAL PROGRAMMING

We will discuss recreational activities in detail under programming. The initial assessment of activities is to determine the programming opportunities that exist for the mentally impaired of varying abilities. To understand the need for recreational development, staff are asked to identify:

> Which clients are involved in everything - participate in at least one or two programs per day.
>
> Which clients are involved in some things - participate in four to seven programs per week.
>
> Which clients are involved in little or nothing - involved in less than three programs per week.

Utilizing recreational activities as part of programming requires a wide variety of activities geared to different levels of functioning. Should those opportunities be limited, then there are few options available to the care team to exhaust, redirect or occupy the time of specific mentally impaired clients.

LIVE ON THE UNIT

One of the best assessment tools that can be implemented is to have one staff member and/or manager live on a unit that houses the mentally impaired clients. (When assessing a facility, I personally will live on the unit for a two day period.) During that time the organizational representative is to participate in everything - meal times with the clients, sitting in the lounge, attending activities, being placed in the tub (with their clothes on). Staff are encouraged to treat the individual as though that person were a client, not changing what they do and how they do it.

The representative is responsible to do a thorough analysis of the pressures encountered by the mentally impaired on that unit. The material generated can be used to develop an educational package for staff, and also to challenge the care team on some of its routines. Of course the staff member conducting this assessment must have a positive rapport with the care team to ensure that caregivers perceive this as a positive experience.

ASSESSING AGGRESSIVE EPISODES

Each aggressive episode, regardless of its severity, must be examined thoroughly. The mentally impaired are communicating through their behavior. The aggressive/violent episode is often a signal to the caregiver that a possible causative factor exists. Until it is resolved, the potential for a recurrence of that behavior is always present.

Whenever an aggressive/violent episode of a mentally impaired client is encountered, the following should be examined:

> Map the client's activity and whereabouts prior to the aggressive/violent episode.
> Identify who was on duty the past sixteen hours to define possible personality conflicts.
> Identify what is different than normal within the environment, the individual's routine, medications used, etc.?
> Identify what was going on around and to the person at that time?
> Determine how the situation could have been handled differently.

The analysis of each aggressive/violent episode must be recorded and then compared. This comparing may uncover a pattern that will lead to preventing the next aggressive response.

SUMMARY

Of all the assessment tools discussed, intuition is probably the most powerful. Some believe that intuition has limited effectiveness in providing useful information. On the contrary, intuition is based on two solid pieces of information:

Experience and Knowing the Person

The first part is experience. No text book, no theory, no academic knowledge is ever thorough enough to truly prepare one for the challenges that this clientele will present. Knowledge provides valuable guidelines and can enhance a person's skills, but it is not enough. The mentally impaired are our teachers. It is the actual contact, the repeated trial and error, the frustrations and rewards encountered that will create an effective *investigative caregiver*. A person who has acquired a "sixth sense." An ability to uncover what needs to be done, not only to prevent Alzheimer's aggression, but to ensure a quality of life.

The second part of intuition is knowledge about the individual client. The longer a caregiver works with the individual, the more that will be learned about the specific needs of that person.

The best assessment source is the direct line caregiver (family, nurse, housekeeper, recreation staff, dietary, etc.). These are the people who possess the ability to define programming needs. If they are skilled investigators, their intuitive ability becomes the key to defining successful programming.

Chapter Six

PROGRAMMING

Programming for the mentally impaired is comprised of an array of options. Each works with some mentally impaired, minimally with others and is totally inappropriate for the remainder. The challenge is in determining which "tool" fits which client at what time. Assessment establishes the need, but defining the right programming is determined often by trial and error. This involves attempting a specific programming option, if it works stay with it, and if it doesn't discard it and try something else. This experimentation is a major part of programming definition for the mentally impaired.

The success of programming depends on the caregiver's ability to be flexible, consistent and creative. The first two terms seem contradictory, yet are quite compatible with each other. Flexibility allows the caregiver to adapt to the needs of the client. Consistency ensures that the effective programming for a specific client is used at all times by all caregivers. In a sense, caregivers need to clone each other. It should not matter whether the client is in contact with one caregiver or another, the approach, expectations, and supports should always be the same.

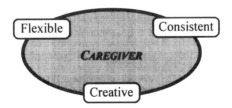

Creativity is being the investigative caregiver - always looking for something more as the vulnerability of the client increases. The care team can never be satisfied with the status quo. The status quo changes as the individual's needs and abilities change. The progressive nature of the disease means that this is a never ending cycle - creativity/ flexibility/consistency.

The three outcomes to programming are:

Divert these are strategies employed during times of distress and are intended to change the client's emotional state by changing the individual's thought process. It is based on a fundamental concept involving the mentally impaired:

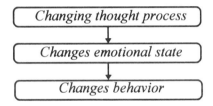

Redirect These tactics remove the individual from the distressor and focus the client's energy elsewhere.

Retract These care strategies remove the distressor and leave the client alone to settle.

Each of these components will be discussed in the following pages.

The term *programming* includes anything and everything that can create any one of these three outcomes. The focus of this chapter is not to identify all of the programming options available. That would be a monumental task. Instead we will concentrate on those programming strategies that specifically apply to aggressive behavior.

When discussing programming, it is important first to define how and why programming is used. Once the programming purpose, response and focus are determined, then the wide range of programming options available will be more apparent.

THE PURPOSE OF PROGRAMMING

The purpose of programming is often misunderstood. Some believe that programming is only successful when it <u>stops</u> a client's aggressive behavior. That belief is in error.

Programming is not intended to stop aggressive behavior.

Its purpose is to make that behavior tolerable to those who must be in contact with the client and to eliminate the possible distressor that is creating it.

To demonstrate the significance of this concept, let us return to the discussion on Care Analysis presented in the previous chapter. The client discussed experienced "aggressive behavior during meal time."

During the first care conference, it was hypothesized that the causative factor may be *bombarding.* Supports were implemented to resolve that issue. Had the aggressive behavior continued after the interventions were realized, then the situation would need to be re-assessed again at another conference. In the next conference the causative factor identified was *inappropriate approach.* It is still possible that those interventions may not be sufficient to eliminate the client's aggressive behavior. The case would need to be examined again, this time to reveal that the *environment* may be a causative factor.

After all of this effort, supports in the area of bombardment, approach and environment may still not stop the client's aggressive behavior. The aggressive episodes may continue regardless of the efforts of the caregiver. The question often asked is - "What is the value of the effort if the behavior does not stop?" The answer is most significant - the value is *quality of life.* The benefits of this analysis and the subsequent programming that is implemented provides for this client the most positive setting given the individual's strengths, limitations and vulnerabilities. That is the mandate of our role.

For some, that may not be enough of a motivation. Then let us look at it another way. Imagine that:

It is known by all caregivers
That bombarding, approach and environment

Are highly sensitive issues for this client/
Regardless of that knowledge,
The necessary supports are not provided consistently/
How much aggression will the caregivers encounter then?

The answer is simple - **lots**.

If the supports are consistently provided in these three areas,
How much aggression will the caregivers encounter then?

The answer now is - **less**.

That is the entire purpose of programming for the mentally impaired. It is not how to stop aggression but how to make it <u>tolerable</u>. That concept is based on a simple fact -

If there is a symptom of the mentally impaired
that can be stopped with something other than medication,
then it is not Alzheimer's that is causing it.

It may at times be impossible to stop a client's behavior through various programming strategies. The success of programming is to lessen the intensity or frequency of that behavior. It is better to have less aggression, than more aggression at any time.

PROGRAMMING FOCUS

Programming is tentacled. It does not just target the client affected, but also those who the behavior may be affecting. On a unit housing many mentally impaired clients, the intense behavioral response of one client can have a domino-effect, creating far-reaching ramifications for the entire unit. Whether that behavior is aggression, wandering, repetitive speech, rummaging and hoarding, etc., there is more that must be examined than just the client in question. In a long term care facility, the programming focus must include four components.

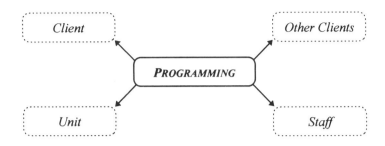

1) Individual Client

We have discussed at length the sensitivity of the mentally impaired to stimuli and how it can initiate an aggressive response. However, there are behaviors that certain mentally impaired clients demonstrate that impact on others, and may not effect them personally. An example is repetitive speech. This is a client who will repeat the same word, phrase or sounds constantly throughout the day. The cause is biological in nature (persistent stimuli). This is an unconscious activity that may exhaust the client, but often does not create any emotional distress for the person doing it. This type of behavior usually stops when the client is distracted (a distraction causes a change in brain wave pattern that overrides the damaged area within the brain).

2) Other Clients

The responsibility of the care team is to identify others on the unit with a low tolerance level for this behavior. Imagine that the client performing the repetitive speech is Mary. A male mentally impaired client (Jack) can only tolerate her repetitive calling out for about forty-five minutes at a time. Unfortunately, routines on the unit are haphazardly scheduled, based either on room location or convenience. The morning progresses as follows:

At 0830 hours, Mary has her morning care
and is in the lounge from 0915 to 1200 hours.
At 0830 Jack attends an activity
and is in the lounge from 0915 to 1200 hours.
By 1000 hours Jack is highly distressed and aggressive.

Schedules and routines are a major programming tool. They can often be used to divert or re-direct. When caregivers do not consciously organize routines and schedules to accommodate potential stressors, then they have lost a valuable aspect of programming. In the above case it is very easy to eliminate the aggressive response of the second client. A *simplistic* alternate schedule is as follows:

> Mary is in the lounge from 0830 hours.
> Jack attends his activity at 0830 hours
>   and returns to the lounge at 915 hours.
> At 1000 hours Mary has her morning care.
> Jack remains in the lounge.
> Mary returns to the lounge at 1045 hours.
> Both clients go for lunch at 1145 hours.

Clients sensitive to the actions or behaviors of other clients must be identified through the process of patterning. The schedules and routines of the day can then be used to break the pattern of behavior.

3) The Unit

The tolerance level of those living on a unit must also be monitored. If after an hour and half of Mary's calling out, a number of clients become distressed, then interventions must be employed at specific times. The schedule presented earlier removes Mary from the unit at 1000 hours, and lunch will break that pattern as well. At other high sensitive times for the unit, she can be easily distracted by simply having tea and toast or a recreational program each hour to hour and half throughout the day. Hence the involvement of family, volunteer and recreational staff, along with Mary's scheduled care becomes an ideal programming package that can break the pattern.

4) Staff

The caregiver cannot be overlooked when defining programming focus. In dealing with any behavior, the caregiver must be asked, "How long can staff handle this behavior?" If the staff generally say, "no more than two hours," then why would any caregiver be assigned to this client for a longer period?

If assigned for a full eight hour shift, there is no question that the patience of even the most dedicated caregiver would be worn thin. Once that occurs, then the caregiver's objectivity and approach could be jeopardized not only with this client, but with every other client that this caregiver contacts.

A unit cannot afford to have its staff lose control. When staff lose control by being placed in an intolerable situation, they lose control with all of the clients they are in contact with. In this situation, two staff may need to be assigned to this client every shift, with each person alternating two hours about. It may influence continuity of care, but at least when staff enter the room after two hours away they are objective and in control.

In the situation where an individual caregiver or just a few have difficulty with a specific behavior, then the need is obvious - training. They require the skills to be able to cope with that behavior.

This four part focus in programming definition must become standardized on any unit, whether the initiating behavior is aggression, loud verbalization, swearing, striking out, etc. When such behaviors occur, specific questions must be asked:

> What is causing the client's behavior, at which times?
> What affect does it have on other clients, at which times?
> What affect does it have on the unit, at which times?
> What affect does it have on staff, at which times?

With this focus, programming is thorough and accurate.

PROGRAMMING RESPONSE

Understanding that programming involves experimentation (trial and error), it is important to define what that means to the client. The response by the client to a specific programming option dictates its appropriateness for this client and determines the impact on other programming strategies. The programming options can include anything

- activities of daily living, visits from family/volunteers, recreational program, etc. There are four different responses to programming:

$\Rightarrow$ *Involved/No change*
$\Rightarrow$ *Involved/Exhausted*
$\Rightarrow$ *Involved/Excited*
$\Rightarrow$ *Involved/Distressed*

Involved/No Change

This is the mentally impaired client who is involved in programming and on completion experiences no change. Take a recreational program such as a bus trip as an example. A client participates and enjoys the activity. On her return to the unit there is no change compared to before she left. She presents the same physical and mental ability as prior to going on the trip.

Involved/Exhausted

This is the mentally impaired client who is involved in programming and on completion is exhausted. This person participated on the bus trip and enjoyed it. Even so, the activity for this client was demanding, both physically and mentally. It tired her out and on return to the unit she needs a rest period before she will regain the same physical and mental ability as prior to going on the trip.

Involved/Excited

This is the mentally impaired client who is involved in programming and on completion is excited. This person participated on the bus trip and enjoyed it. However, the activity stirred many positive memories for this individual and peaked his energy level. On return to the unit it takes time for him to settle and present the same physical and mental ability as prior to going on the trip.

Involved/Distressed

This is the mentally impaired client who is involved in programming and on completion is distressed. This person participated and enjoyed the activity. On her return she is distressed for a considerable period of time after the activity. She is hypersensitive to any further stimuli, which increases the risk for an aggressive response. The probability of her being sedated as a result is high. For this client, this activity is considered a *taboo*. Taboos are programming options that are tolerated poorly by specific mentally impaired clients. Even though the person may be involved and enjoy that activity, *the negative consequences of the activity outweigh the benefits.* The client, through her behavior, is communicating that she cannot handle the stimuli and should not be involved.

We need to examine each of these responses in order to demonstrate programming direction. The first and last response are obvious. The first response *involved/no change* means that the client should be encouraged to attend that activity. The second response, *involved/distress* is also obvious. The person cannot handle the activity as it is, and therefore should not attend until it is adapted or should be provided an alternate activity. It is the second and third response that can stir considerable controversy.

Some caregivers may attempt to restrict the client's involvement because she returns either exhausted or excited.

When the client returns from an activity exhausted, these caregivers will justify barring her involvement the next time on the grounds that on return she will not complete her care (i.e. needs to be fed, instead of feeding herself).

When the client is involved and returns excited, some caregivers believe that she shouldn't be allowed to go, because on return she will not settle right away and that makes it difficult to perform her care.

Being barred from attending an activity for either of these reasons, demonstrates the care philosophy of the staff and organization concerned - they are a passive care setting and care oriented rather than client centered. In this type of living environment, the only time a mentally impaired client is allowed to attend an activity is when it does not affect the care routine.

A quality care setting and a client centered philosophy will see the situation differently. They are willing to adapt to the client. When the person returns from any activity exhausted or excited, they will assist the individual with any task or allow the person "to wind down" before introducing anything else. Either way the care routine is adapted to the client.

Many are surprised at the emphasis of scheduling activities and tasks as major components of programming. Programming does have special tools, but much of programming centers around existing tools and how they are used. There are many quality care settings that have few formalized programming options available, but those settings allow their staff the freedom to use what they have to divert, re-direct or retract.

This concept of client response needs to be taken further. The dynamics just described reflect the team dynamics of a unit. In certain care settings (usually those of a passive care focus), it seems as though each department is like an "island," working independently of each other with limited communication.

For an example, the recreation staff, volunteers or family take a mentally impaired client out to an activity. They are pleased that the client participated and enjoyed the event. Unfortunately, there is minimal communication from nursing staff that the client was highly distressed and aggressive for hours after he returned to the unit. Therefore, the nursing staff do not send that client to the next activity or possibly any related activity for fear that he may become distressed again (remember the example from the case in chapter two - doctors order "To be restricted from all activities").

Programming is not defined by individuals. It is defined by the care team. All parties need to know the consequences, discuss how the situation can be handled differently, determine what alternative activity can be attempted or ways of supporting the individual during those activities. Each member of that team has an expertise that is crucial in identifying the pieces of the puzzle needed to assist the client. The information and knowledge of one member, in combination with another, builds a programming package for each client.

Now that the foundation for programming has been defined, let us examine some programming options as they apply to the concepts of programming purpose, response and focus.

> **Retract** *these are strategies that remove the distressor and leave the client alone to settle.*

There are situations in dealing with a distressed mentally impaired client when the best strategy is to retract or back off. Retracting involves removing the stressor and ensuring that the client is not subjected to any further stimuli for a specified period of time. For some mentally impaired clients, simply being left alone after the stressor is removed is sufficient. For other mentally impaired clients, it requires removing the individual completely from contact with others for a period of time.

STRESSOR ELIMINATION PROCESS

We have identified a number of environmental stimuli that can distress the mentally impaired - fire drills, visitors, noise level, decor, etc. The Stressor Elimination Process is intended to control that stimuli. To demonstrate ways to control environmental stimuli let us examine the impact of a *chaotic event*.

Chaotic Events

Chaotic events are events that occur outside the norm of the day's routine, such as fire drills, repairing alarm systems, PA feedback, structural repairs (fixing plumbing, walls, ceilings, etc.), renovations, open house, and so on. This type of stimuli is usually quite dramatic - loud enough to be heard throughout the unit and creating multiple stimuli at one time. The mentally impaired are unable to relate to a chaotic event for a number of reasons:

- loss of analytical ability prevents them from determining what it is.
- increased sensitivity to bombarding decreases their ability to relate to what is experienced.
- lack of recall results in their forgetting where they are and who/what may be making the commotion.
- sensitivity to stimuli means that they are easily overwhelmed by the intensity of the experience.
- obscurity of the activity results in their inability to define its specific location or direction.

Probably one of the most chaotic events to occur on any unit is a fire drill. Without warning alarm bells sound, staff rush about, doors are closed, clients are corralled to a specific location, etc. After a few moments of this hyperactivity, staff will be told that the drill is over. It may be over for the staff, but it is not necessarily over for their mentally impaired clients. Even though a silent alarm is best (a fire drill without the bells), the rest of the stimuli is still in place and can create similar dynamics. The response by the mentally impaired to a fire drill is varied.

⇒ Some mentally impaired clients will experience no change after a fire drill. They will be able to resume their normal routine without any difficulty.

⇒ Others will find the demands of the fire drill to be exhausting. They will need to be removed from any further stimuli for a period of time.

⇒ Others will be excited by the fire drill. They will become vocal, wander or attempt to leave the building. They will need time to settle before they can return to their normal routine.

⇒ Still others will become distressed by the drill, hypersensitive to any further stimuli. They will need to be left alone for a considerable period before they can return to their normal routine.

It is interesting when some caregivers attempt to resume the scheduled routine of a mentally impaired client (i.e. bath, recreational activity, etc.) only minutes after a fire drill. Normally these clients would be cooperative with that scheduled activity. Those responding to the drill in the latter three ways cannot tolerate any further stimuli. Introducing any further demands on these clients after a fire drill only results in their becoming agitated. These normally tolerated activities now become circumstantial episodes, elevating anxiety to a panic state. A simple rule on a unit that houses the mentally impaired is:

After a chaotic event
all programming will be delayed for one hour
for some mentally impaired clients.
Others will require all but basic care stopped
for the remainder of the day.

The response by some caregivers to this requirement is always fascinating. It is commonly heard - "We don't have time for that." Time is not the issue. Time is a constant. It will be invested no matter what is done. The differences in approach is problem solving versus crisis intervention.

There are only two options after a chaotic event. One is to wait for certain clients to settle before resuming the care routine. The other is to resume the care routine regardless of what is going on around or to the client. To give a mentally impaired client a bath shortly after a fire drill has the following results:

⇒ requires two staff instead of one.
⇒ the client will fight staff down the hall.
⇒ fight them in the tub.
⇒ all three will have a bath.
⇒ she will fight them out of the tub and to get dressed.
⇒ she will be highly agitated for a considerable period of time afterwards.

Not only is the event detrimental to the client, it is poor time management on the part of the caregivers. Being able to adapt to circumstances such as these is a true test of the investigative caregiver (flexible/consistent/creative) and a quality care setting.

Unit Monitor

A unit that houses the mentally impaired must be a controlled environment. This does not imply that family and visitors should be restricted. However, tour groups, activities, other departments on the unit, schedules, etc. must be monitored and at times restricted. When the environment is not controlled, aggressive behavior is a common occurrence.

A successful programming option for any unit housing this type of clientele is to assign one staff member each shift as a Unit Monitor. A Unit Monitor is given a red name tag (an alternate staff member takes the role during that person's lunch and coffee breaks). The Unit Monitor is responsible to monitor and control the noise level of the unit. That means that nothing is to come on the unit outside of the regular daily routines without checking with the Unit Monitor first. The Unit Monitor, along with feedback from the rest of the team, will determine the appropriateness and outcome of that event.

Whether it is a tour group, recreation program, floor polisher, maintenance staff repairing a toilet, etc. these cannot be done without consideration to those living on that unit. A sign can be placed at the entrance to the unit that anyone entering the unit (other than family, visitors and the normal daily movement of staff) must please check with the Unit Monitor first.

The responsibility of the Unit Monitor is to determine the appropriateness of what is to occur, given what is happening on the unit at that time. The Unit Monitor must have the authority to request anyone entering the unit to delay what is required if it is believed that the unit is not equipped or prepared to handle the chaos that can result. An alternate time needs to be arranged when the care team is able to handle the individual(s) who may not cope well with the stimuli.

An example is a tour group of six professionals wanting to tour the unit. The Unit Monitor could:

- identify the best time for the tour group to arrive on this unit.
- request two at a time to tour, to decrease the stimuli.
- encourage the tour group to wait for a period until the clients are distracted with an activity.
- request that the tour not occur at this time (if the circumstances on the unit are already chaotic).

The freedom for the caregivers to have this type of control is the true sign of a client centered care philosophy. It is the clients who are considered first, beyond what the organization requires.

This unit, its clients and its staff cannot experience surprises. The Unit Monitor is responsible to assist those individuals coming on the unit who do not understand the special needs of this clientele. The Unit Monitor can then determine if their going on the unit is appropriate at that time, instruct them on what to do and what not to do, where to do it, who to watch for, what to say, and then prepare the rest of the team for the consequences.

The Unit Monitor has another responsibility, to monitor the noise and activity level of the unit's daily routines. There are times when there is just too much going on all at once. During periods when everything seems to be happening, the care team needs to be instructed to stop their schedule and decrease the noise level. They need to focus on the clients to decrease the distress created by the commotion occurring at that time.

The comment from some is again "That is impossible. We will never get anything done." In a passive care setting, where there are no environmental controls, they may be right. Such a setting is generally in chaos. Taking time to allow the clients to settle would need to occur so frequently that little could get done. In a quality care setting however, such chaos is unusual. Their routines are client centered, sensitive to the vulnerability of the client. Like a fire drill, they know that their activity level can have as much influence on the distress level of their clients. They place the client above the care routine.

Some are surprised at the emphasis on environmental control as a part of programming. The rational is clear. When external factors are not controlled - schedules and routines, other clients, environment, etc. - the effectiveness of specific intervention strategies that distract or redirect are handicapped. It is similar to the rebound effect of medication described in chapter three. If the causative factor is still in place, no matter what interventions are employed, they will eventually lose their effectiveness until the distressor is eliminated.

When a mentally impaired client does not respond well to a specific programming option (divert, redirect or retract), what is the reason? - the programming option is inappropriate or the external factor is diluting its effectiveness. Once external factors are controlled, the response by the mentally impaired to the majority of programming options becomes much more effective.

Energy Conservation

Many caregivers know the benefits of a short rest period or nap in the morning and another in the afternoon for certain mental impaired clients. Rest or nap periods remove a mentally impaired client from the accumulation of stressors, decreases anxiety, and provides the individual the opportunity to recharge physical and mental energies in preparation for the next barrage of stimuli.

Retracting or backing off is a static process. For some mentally impaired it is all that is needed to decrease their distress and prevent aggression. For others, more direct programming options such as diverting and redirecting are needed to create the desired outcome.

Divert   *these are strategies employed during times of distress intended to change the clients emotional state by changing the individual's thought process.*

Diverting relates to a significant concept that applies to the mentally impaired - the mentally impaired have limited recall due to short term memory loss. Changing the individual's thought process will distract the person from whatever is distressing him. However, if the negative emotion associated with that distressor is not negated, then the person will still be aggressive. If the past memory recalled can hook a positive emotion, then the distressor is not only forgotten, but the negative emotion is replaced as well.

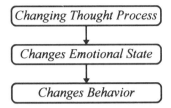

Hence changing the thought process can eliminate distress and prevent aggression from occurring. However, the basic concept about programming effectiveness still exists even with diverting tactics. With diverting it:

⇒ *works with some mentally impaired.*
⇒ *minimally with others.*
⇒ *totally inappropriate for the remainder.*

There are many programming options that fit the criteria as distracters:

1) Family

The presence of family commonly has associated with it positive past memories. In many instances, a mentally impaired client will soon forget what was distressing, and smile at the presence of a family member.

Unfortunately, without direction, family often visit at inappropriate times. Many families believe that it is best to visit when the unit is quiet and to leave when the unit is busy. They feel that when the unit is busy they may be "in the way." On the contrary, with this type of client it is best that family visit when the unit is busy and leave when it is quiet.

When the unit is quiet staff can focus their attention on the clients in need and divert or redirect them as required. When the unit is busy, staff are too occupied to adequately attend to those clients. If possible, family visiting should not be haphazardly scheduled. Their visits are a valuable part of programming. Once a behavior is defined (through patterning), then family must not only be given direction on the best times to visit, but also on the things to do during those visits. If family perceives that their only role is to carry on a conversation with a mom/dad, then the visits can have limited benefit and family will easily become frustrated. Family need to learn how to divert or redirect mom/dad during the visit.

2) Cue Words

These are very valuable if they can be discovered. Cue words are words that will *immediately* snap a mentally impaired client into past positive memory. An example is a client who always discusses her husband (Joe). When she becomes distressed, she need only be asked, "What would **Joe** think about that?" The husband's name is accentuated by tone and a <u>slightly</u> louder volume. When a cue word is used, it is possible to see the client's thought process shift. She will pause, look away, smile and may begin talking about her husband. The distressor has been forgotten, her emotional state and behavior changed. There are many examples of cue words:

Past History	Cue Word (**Bolded**)
Past farmer always talking about the horses.	"I wonder how the **horses** are doing on a rainy day like this?"
Mother always talking about her children (Elizabeth & John)	"I haven't seen your daughter **Elizabeth** or your son **John** for awhile."
Previous school teacher	"The kids are in **school** today. I wonder what they are doing?"

One example that demonstrated the value of a cue word involved a mentally impaired client who was an avid fisherman. He always talked about "the big one." During contact with him on a specific occasion, he was highly agitated. He was simply asked, "What lure is the best to catch **the big one**?" He smiled and walked away. There was no further conversation. His emotional state changed along with his behavior as he thought about "the big one."

3) Topics of Conversation

Unlike cue words, topics of conversation do not have the same *immediate* effect. When a cue word is not available, focusing on certain topics and expanding them will often draw a mentally impaired client back into a past memory. The more the person recalls that memory, the more a change in her emotional state and behavior will be noticed. Family assessment must include asking - What did your family member like to talk about in the past? What does she like to talk about now?

4) Pictures or Keepsake Items

At distressful times, directing the attention of the mentally impaired to pictures of family members or keepsake items (comforter from home, personal chair, etc.) become valuable distracters. They may draw the client back to a past positive thought process and elicit a positive emotional response to counter the distressor experienced.

5) Music

"Old fashioned music" is often an effective distracter for many mentally impaired clients, whether through a sing-a-long, record player or radio. The music must be from their past (1930 to 1950). (You know you have the right music playing when young staff hate it.) However it must be remembered that music is minimally tolerated by some mentally impaired and perceived as noise by others.

Timing is the key. If music is always on, cr on during stress saturated times (meal time), then it will become a distressor for most mentally impaired. If used based on need, it is effective.

Singing or humming while toileting, dressing or bathing a client will have a similar effect. If the task is difficult for this person to perform, then distracting the individual becomes effective. The task is done without the person's attention being focused on it.

6) Recreational Activities

There are a variety of activities that illicit positive past emotions. They include such familiar events as baking, eating, having a glass of beer, gardening, social activities (tea), crafts, etc.

7) Sensory Stimulation

These tools are used to stimulate the senses - touch, smell, sight and/or taste and are used to subsequently recall past events. They can be used very effectively as a distracter if they relate to the client's past history. Some units have developed what are called theme boxes. These are permanently established boxes with specific items related to specific themes that can be used at any time for the appropriate client:

Past History	Contents of Theme Box
carpenter	wood, sandpaper, small antique tools
sewer	wool, thread, fabric
gardener	seeds, dried flowers, gardening hat, flower book
fisherman	fishing line, reel, fishing hat, fishing magazine
golfer	golf balls, tees, golfing pictures

Distracters are effective programming tools. They are client specific. Knowledge of the client's past history is key to ensuring the success of these strategies.

> **Redirect** These tactics remove the individual from the distressor and focus the client's energy elsewhere.

When a mentally impaired client is distressed, redirecting is intended to decrease anxiety, and focus the stressful energy created by the distressor in a more positive direction. The rational for these strategies is related to the physiological effect a distressor creates.

At a time of stress, the person's state of readiness is heightened to fight what is experienced. Simply using a diverting tactic may not be sufficient for some mentally impaired. Although the distressor may be forgotten and the emotions changed, the person may still be hypersensitive to stimuli and stress. Unless the energy produced by the experience is redirected or exhausted, then it will result in a negative outcome.

Most redirecting activities have many functions besides focusing and exhausting energy. They also:

- give a sense of purpose
- occupy time
- are enjoyable
- will help the person sleep at night

1) Chores

Activities such as cleaning table tops, assisting with laundry, sweeping, etc. do not have to be learned. They relate well to the individual's past history. It is common to have certain mentally impaired clients initiate these on their own.

2) Walking

This is probably one of the most effective ways to redirect energy. The goal of a walking program for certain mentally impaired clients during times of distress is to identify the furthest and fastest the person can safely go.

3) Activities of Daily Living

As demonstrated earlier, the scheduling of activities of daily living tasks such as bathing, dressing, meal time, toileting, etc. can be used to redirect energy and remove the person from a specific distressor.

4) Relaxation Techniques

It is always a pleasure to watch skilled caregivers in action, who have a natural talent for working with the mentally impaired elderly. Often when contacting certain clients, these caregivers will instinctively begin stroking the person's hair, hand or massaging their back. This is a successful technique for some mentally impaired.

When these caregivers are asked why they approach those clients in that manner, they will often say "I don't know, it just works." Usually they intuitively have identified the pre-emptive cueing (the face) to indicate that the client is stressed and have employed a basic relaxation technique. In actual, fact the caregiver in that situation is decreasing the client's tension (energy) level even before any further demands are placed on the individual.

There are many relaxation techniques that are employed formally with the mentally impaired - back or foot massage, hot baths, deep breathing exercises (if the client is able to follow direction).

DRUG UTILIZATION STRATEGIES

You will notice that drug utilization is the last programming option discussed. At times, medication for aggressive behavior is needed as a stop gap measure until another strategy can be employed to eliminate the distressor and decrease the aggressive behavior.

The difference in medication use as a programming option is that it is not reactive - waiting for the behavior to occur and then administering the sedation. Instead medication is used proactively. The person's worst time of the day is identified through patterning. When no programming strategy has been identified as yet to lessen the distress at that time, then administering a mild sedation an hour to an hour and half before is effective. The intention is to help the client over the distressful period, even though the cause has not been defined and other strategies are not as yet successful (divert, redirect or retract).

However, the investigative caregiver does not stop looking for an alternative to medication. The care team knows that this person's abilities, limitations and vulnerabilities will change over time. At some point the need for that medication will have eliminated itself and the drug can be discontinued.

SUMMARY

Watching a skilled craftsperson ply his/her art is quite a thrill. Whether it is a professional artist, carpenter or sculptor, the person makes it look so easy. They seem to know just when to use the right tool, how to handle it in a manner that brings the object to life. In actual fact, for most craftspeople it took years of learning, practicing and experimenting to develop their skills to that level. Now it is second nature and can be done with the least effort and thought.

It is always amazing how some will believe that what has been discussed on assessment and programming is too difficult, too complex, too time consuming, too . . . Yet others see it as a challenge, exciting and rewarding. The strategies identified to divert, redirect or retract require the skill of a craftsperson. Through practice, knowledge and experimentation the investigative caregiver knows just when to use what tool, for what effect, for how long, to be able to return quality life back to the client under their care.

There are two remaining areas that must be examined before we can bring this to a close - approaching the client and what is needed to meet the challenge.

Chapter Seven

THE CONTROLLING APPROACH

Imagine:

>You are sitting in a chair
>You do not know me/
>I approach you
>While standing over top of you
>You hear "Tho vou stas deau kau tho da vadvron?"/
>I then grab your right arm and try to lift you from your chair/

>What would be your response?

Change that scenario:

>You are sitting in a chair
>You do not know me
>I approach you/
>Crouch down along side of you at eye level/
>Gently touch your arm/
>Smile, and say in a soft voice
>"Tho vou stas deau kau tho da vadvron?"/
>I lightly touch your elbow
>To assist you to stand/

>What is the chance of your cooperating?

There is no doubt that in either situation you would be suspicious. In the first your reaction would likely be to fight. In the second you may be cautiously cooperative.

Persons who have lost recent memory and analytical ability experience a common problem - every stimuli, face, or noise has to be analyzed constantly. This need limits the ability to respond to information quickly enough in order to react appropriately. Of all that has been discussed to this point on preventing Alzheimer's Aggression, there is nothing that seems to be more crucial than rapport or trust. Rapport, or the immediate feelings associated with the initial contact, will dictate the outcome of any interaction.

The mentally impaired find themselves continuously being guided about by people they do not know. Therefore, the first seconds of contact determines if that person should cautiously cooperate, fight or flight. Some mentally impaired establish rapport with others quickly. They cooperate willingly when moved from one location to another, from one task to another. They seem to have unlimited trust in others. There are other mentally impaired clients who need that rapport established on each contact. In fact, if rapport is not established, it is these individuals who will commonly become aggressive.

Rapport with the mentally impaired cannot be taken lightly. It can be made or broken within the first few seconds of contact. Our actions are often faster than the mentally impaired client's ability to analyze them. Subsequently, on first contact, speech comprehension by the mentally impaired is limited. Asking the question, "Do you have to go to the bathroom?" may sound no different than saying, "Tho vou stas deau kau tho da vadvron?" When a person cannot remember where she is or who the people are around her, then the cueing provided dictates how to respond.

This is not a conscious process. The reactions of the mentally impaired are not dictated by their ability to analyze the situation. Their cognitive ability is too limited to perform such a complex task. Instead they are influenced more by the emotional state created by any stimuli. If anxiety is not elevated, then the chances of responding appropriately are good. If anxiety is pushed to a panic state by the inappropriateness of the approach, then the only reaction is to fight, flight or withdraw.

Understanding what differentiates those who work well with the mentally impaired, from those who do not, has always been a challenge. Observing scores of caregivers caring for numerous mentally impaired clients has uncovered a significant fact - how the caregiver approaches the client has a dramatic influence on the outcome of that contact.

In one situation two caregivers were observed approaching a mentally impaired client who had a history of aggressive behavior. The male client was sitting in a chair in the lounge. Standing four feet away from him, one of the caregiver's stated, "Luigi, it is time for your shave."

The caregivers appeared as though they were choreographed. They proceeded to walk around either side of the client. Once behind him, they were oblivious from his view. Without warning, both caregivers simultaneously placed a hand on each of the client's shoulders, and the other hand on each of his wrists in order to lift him from the chair. Luigi immediately began to fight.

The caregivers were stopped and asked, "If this man did not have a history of being aggressive, would you have approached him differently?" One of them stated, "If we weren't so afraid of being kicked, there would only need to be one of us and we would have approached him from the front. But when you do that, it is too easy for him to hit you." Their approach only initiated what they were trying to stop.

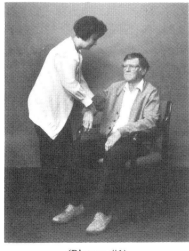

(Picture #1)

In the first few seconds of contact, the initial actions of the caregiver can be too fast and abrupt. Without the appropriate cueing, the client can be immediately put on guard. (Picture #1). When verbal comprehension is lost, the only way the mentally impaired can react is by responding to the facial expression, posture and mannerism of the caregiver. When the mentally impaired are approached in the manner depicted in the picture, they are not given:

- any warning of the action being taken.
- the opportunity to see the face of the individual who has made contact.
- the time to process the actions of the individual.
- the support to understand what is being requested.
- the ability to adapt to the multiple stimuli occurring in the short period available.
- the opportunity to focus on the task at hand.

Within seconds of the caregiver's contact, a mentally impaired client is required to change his thought process from whatever is occurring in his mind to determining who and what that person wants. Without that ability, the person feels further out of control, and anxiety is peaked to a panic state. The basis for the aggressive cycle begins.

Those caregivers who have a problem with the mentally impaired demonstrate two significant limitations in their approach.

1) The caregiver has an approach that intensifies the client's anxiety level.

2) The caregiver is not in control of the situation and is usually at risk.

Those who encounter significant resistance, aggression or violent behavior from the mentally impaired can often initiate it by their approach. Likewise, when aggressive behavior does occur, they seem less able to deal with it effectively to bring the situation under control and prevent themselves or others from being injured.

On the other hand, when the mentally impaired encounter a more supportive approach, they have an opportunity to react to the facial expression, body movements and gestures of the caregiver. When this cueing is direct and positive, the client has a feeling of being more in control. This decreases the need to become resistive or aggressive.

The effective caregiver usually experiences little resistive or aggressive behavior and the times when it does occur, the outcome is often very different for two reasons:

1) The initial physical approach is in a manner that communicates trust (rapport enhancement).

2) When the client reacts in a violent/aggressive manner, the caregiver is able to control the situation (controlling approach).

Rapport enhancement and control are key aspects of preventing and dealing with aggression behavior.

THE NEED TO BE IN CONTROL

No caregiver should ever place themselves in contact with a mentally impaired client believing that the potential for that person to become aggressive does not exist.

The philosophy when working with the mentally impaired is to **expect the unexpected**. Just when you think you know what that person is going to do, there is always the possibility that he will change it.

The mentally impaired are reactive to situations based on how they perceive them. No matter how much we attempt to understand what the world of the mentally impaired may be like, we will never be able to predict it fully. Any caregiver who believes she knows exactly how a mentally impaired client may respond in any given situation is deceiving herself. That perception leads to crisis intervention. It is a philosophy that simply waits for something to happen before steps are taken, the results of which usually are detrimental for both the mentally impaired client and the caregiver.

The effective caregiver attempts to prevent situations from occurring, not deal with them after they have happened.

It is essential that the caregiver is in control each time she is in contact with a mentally impaired client.

In *many* cases when a mentally impaired client has injured a caregiver, it was the staff member who contributed to the result. This is not to say that staff are to blame for the consequences. If they are not specifically trained on how to effectively deal with this type of client, then they are at risk for any possible consequence.

In one example where a staff member was seriously injured by a mentally impaired client, it was discovered that the caregiver walked right into the problem. The potentially aggressive client was in one chair (client 1) and another client was in the other chair, both located in the corner of the room.

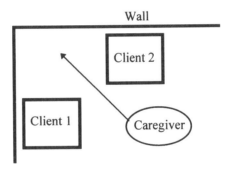

The caregiver stepped into the corner, between the two chairs. She stood above the client (Client 1), to his left side (he was right handed). Without any further warning, she reached for his arm to stand him up. As soon as he stood, he turned towards her. He blocked her into the corner and began striking her. It wasn't until another staff member stepped in and pulled the client away, was she able to free herself. In this instance, the caregiver neither established rapport with the client nor was in control of the situation.

An effective approach must enhance rapport and allow the caregiver to maintain control. The following discusses the Controlling

Approach as it applies to the client who is sitting, standing or lying in bed.

THE CONTROLLING APPROACH

When approaching a right handed client (Picture #2), the caregiver must:

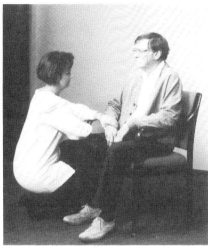

(Picture #2)

1) Approach from the right side.
2) Move any chair or obstacle away from the client's right side.
3) Crouch down below eye level.
4) Place the left hand lightly on the client's right wrist, the right elbow lightly on the client's right knee, right leg against the clients right leg.
5) Keep your body away from the client.

Let us examine each of these to understand their benefits and the outcome.

1) Approach from the dominant side.

There is one question that must be asked about every mentally impaired client:

Which is that person's dominant side, right or left?

If the person is right handed, then one must always approach from the right side. The dominant side is:

- where any reflex action will occur.
- the side where the person is most comfortable.

162

- the side that has the most control, coordination and strength.
- where the person will generally strike first.

Due to the loss of analytical ability by the mentally impaired, their tendency is to respond by reflex in most situations. It is the dominant side of the body from which that reflex action will occur.

Try the following:

Reach out and pick up an object.

Go ahead, nobody is watching you.

If you are right handed, you probably reached for the object using your right hand. Even if that object was located on the left side of your body, you still used your right hand.

You reacted by reflex. It required no thought to determine which hand to use. Furthermore, if you were to strike someone, it would probably be with your dominant hand. It is that side of your body that has the greatest coordination and strength.

The same is true for the mentally impaired. They will *generally* strike from their dominant side. It is a reflex response that requires no analytical thought. If the caregiver is in control of that side of the body, then she is best able to deal with an aggressive or violent response.

Try the following task:

Using your dominant hand only (right hand if you are right hand dominant) take this book and leaf through ten pages. Separate each page one from the other.

Go ahead, give it a try!

Using your non-dominant hand only (left hand if you are right hand dominant) repeat the same task. Take this book and leaf through ten pages again. Separate each page one from the other.

Go ahead, you have come this far, why stop now?

You will notice that using your non-dominant hand was probably uncomfortable, awkward and required considerable thought. Now take this one step further. Imagine that you lost over 50% of your muscle strength and coordination.

What would that do to your abilities on the dominant side of your body?

What would that do to your abilities on the non-dominant side of your body?

There is no question that the non-dominant side of your body would be even more awkward and difficult to use. This puts further reliance on the dominant side when you require any quick movement with little thought. The same becomes true for the mentally impaired.

Progressive apraxia results in the loss of coordination and muscle strength. Even though the dominant side is affected, it is the non-dominant side that will experience the greatest loss in functioning. This results in the non-dominant side having less reaction time and requiring too much thought to perform the same task as the dominant side.

Approaching from the dominant side not only ensures that the caregiver is in control, but it also enhances rapport. This can be easily demonstrated by simply comparing these dynamics to something more familiar.

You are required to assist a stroke victim to stand. She is paralyzed on the left side of her body .

Which side of the client would you position yourself to assist her - the side that is paralyzed or the side that has the greatest strength and ability?

Undoubtedly, you would assist the client on the side where she has the greatest strength and ability. The same support is needed for the mentally impaired. Approaching the person on the dominant side gives the client better control and a feeling of being more secure.

Assisting from the dominant side allows the client to use the side of the body where he has the greatest coordination, strength and balance. This makes situations less threatening, increasing his willingness to cooperate and decreasing his need to resist or fight.

Determining which side is the client's dominant side can be made easy for the care team. It is simply defining for all caregivers that the client's dominant side is the person's right side unless told differently. Only a small percentage of the population is left handed.

2) *Move any chair or obstacle on the client's right side out of the way.*

Moving obstacles from the client's dominant side encourages rapport enhancement.

⇒ The client's reflex response will be to turn to his dominant side.
⇒ The caregiver can get in close enough to make the gentle touch.
⇒ The caregiver is not hidden from view (too far to his side) or intimidating (directly in front).
⇒ The client feels less threatened by the caregiver's presence.

Removing obstacles also ensures control. When obstacles are removed, it allows the caregiver the opportunity to react should the client become aggressive or violent. That requires a chair next to the client to be removed before the client is assisted to stand.

Seating within the environment cannot be haphazardly arranged. Leaving access to the client's dominant side must be considered when seating the client in the dining room or when placing furniture in the client's room. This approach is no different than seating a stroke victim who is paralyzed on the left side of her body. That person would not be seated with her right side to the wall. It would make it too difficult and unsafe to lift her when such an obstacle is present.

No matter what precautions are taken, there will always be exceptions. Undoubtedly there will be times when obstacles cannot be moved or the person cannot be approached from the dominant side. In those cases, the caregiver must be flexible and adapt to the needs of the moment. If the client must be approached from the non-dominant side, then it should be a mirroring of how to approach from the dominant side - obstacles moved away, left elbow on left knee, right hand on left wrist, body away from the client. It is important to stress that when approaching from the non-dominant side, the client requires more support and allowed a longer time to respond.

3) *Crouch below eye level.*

You will notice (Picture #2, page 162) that the caregiver has positioned herself below the client's eye level. This is done intentionally.

Try the following if you can find someone to cooperate (even though they may think you are a little strange).

Ask someone to stand over you while you are sitting in a chair.
Ask that person to face you at eye level.
Then ask that person to crouch down below eye level.

You will notice a significant difference. In the first two situations, you will feel as though the other person has the control. In the last, it is you who will feel in control.

Most are aware that standing above a person and looking down is threatening. Face-to-face at eye level is better, but it can still be quite intimidating. Positioning below eye level has a significant advantage. It is highly communicative, giving the mentally impaired the feeling of being in control. That in turn prevents the client's anxiety from elevating.

4) *Left hand lightly on the client's right wrist, right elbow lightly on the client's right knee, right leg against the clients right leg.*

The light physical touch creates rapport enhancement.

> ⇒ The person immediately does not feel threatened.
> ⇒ The touch also attracts his attention and encourages eye contact.
> ⇒ Eye contact initiates the necessary thought process to respond to your actions.
> ⇒ He has an opportunity to read the caregiver's facial expression.

This manner of approach ensures that the client's anxiety level is not affected by the approach.

This positioning also controls the dominant side should the person strike.

> ⇒ Keeping the leg next to the client's leg prevents him from kicking.
> ⇒ Keeping the elbow lightly on the client's knee warns of a possible kick and allows the caregiver to restrict the movement should he attempt it.

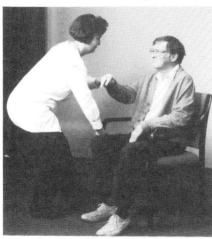

(Picture #3)

> ⇒ The left hand on the right wrist controls his hand should he strike.

Due to the client's limited analytical ability, he will not perceive the light touch on his right wrist and the elbow on his knee as restraining. If he attempts to strike, it will *usually* be from his dominant side. As soon as he raises his right hand to strike, it can easily be deflected and the staff member can back away,

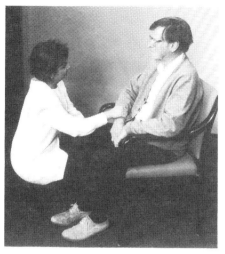

(Picture #4)

(picture #3) employing other strategies in preparation for approaching him again.

It is important that the right hand remain free in order to react in this manner. Some caregivers will have a tendency to place their right elbow on the person's knee and right hand on the person's wrist, leaving their left hand free. (Picture #4) The difficulty with this position is that the caregiver must remove her right hand to deflect a strike from the client's left hand. In doing so, she has let go of his dominant side. The client can easily respond by raising his right hand to strike again. She is no longer in control of the situation.

It is important to note that the caregiver's body is parallel to the client, and off to the side. In this way one cannot be kicked and the caregiver can easily step back if necessary.

It is obvious that the caregiver should never crouch down in front of the client. Placing oneself in front of the client's feet only invites disaster.

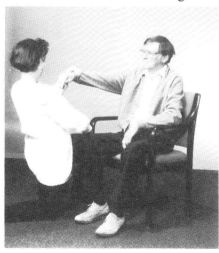

(Picture #5)

There is a tendency by some caregivers to place one knee down on the floor. This position impedes the ability of the caregiver to react if the client does strike. (Picture #5) If the caregiver needs to move out of the way, she is caught. When she attempts to pull back, she will be off balance and unable to stand up. The client can then grab or strike with his left hand.

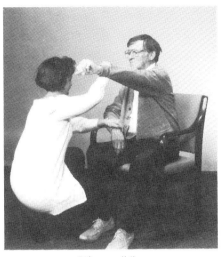

(Picture #6)

5) *Body kept away from the client.*

Keeping the body away from the client makes the caregiver less intimidating, and the client does not feel as though he is being encroached upon. That can increase the immediate rapport experienced by the contact.

It is important to emphasize that the possibility of the client striking with his non-dominant hand is always present. Remember, that successfully working with the mentally impaired requires one to *expect the unexpected*. The caregiver must be in control no matter what occurs. This requires the caregiver to be attentive in every exchange. If the client does strike with his left hand, the distance from the body increases the reaction time available for the caregiver to respond. This allows the caregiver to use her left arm to block or deflect the blow from the client's left hand. (Picture #6)

Even if the person does swing up with his left hand, the caregiver is sitting at the outer range of the blow. In order for the client to extend his reach, he must move his shoulder forward. (Picture #7) That would change his center of gravity and put him off balance, decreasing the likelihood of that occurring.

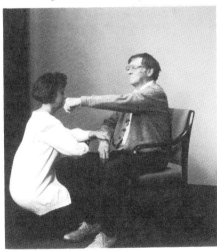

(Picture #7)

SUMMARY: APPROACHING A CLIENT WHO IS SITTING

If a client is right hand dominant, the following summary applies:

Controlling Approach	Cautions
1. Approach from the dominant side	If unable to approach from the dominant side, mirror the controlling approach to the non-dominant side, providing more time and support for the person to respond.
2. Move any chair or obstacle away from the client's dominant side.	Don't sit the client or place furniture haphazardly, without giving consideration to the client's dominant side.
3. Crouch down below eye level.	Do not stand above or at eye level to the client.
4. Place the left hand lightly on the client's right wrist, the right elbow lightly on the client's right knee, right leg against the client's right leg.	Do not place the knee on the floor. Do not place the right hand on the wrist and right elbow on the client's knee. Do not crouch in front of the client.
5. Keep the body away from the client.	Do not move in close.

Always be attentive. There is never a guarantee how a mentally impaired client may respond. There is never that degree of predictability. No approach is foolproof. There is always a degree of risk. Use your judgment to determine what is safe. In unique situations where the caregiver is unsure of how to approach the client, it is the caregiver's responsibility to get direction from the care team, and then in turn from a skilled professional.

THE STEP PROCESS APPROACH

In actual fact even the approach just discussed may be too much or too fast for some mentally impaired clients. When a caregiver is asked the best way to approach a certain mentally impaired client, it is not uncommon to hear "You cannot move in too quickly on that client or she will become aggressive." They have learned that the client needs even more preparation for contact.

The step process approach begins four feet from the client. The goal is to seek eye contact before moving closer. This can be accomplished by calling the client's name. It may be necessary to move to the side in the direction of the client's gaze or crouch down if the client is looking down at the floor. Once eye contact is established, the client has then initiated the needed thought process to prepare for the caregiver's approach.

SITTING WITH A CLIENT

(Picture # 8) It is amazing to watch individuals approach a mentally impaired client in the manner depicted in the picture.

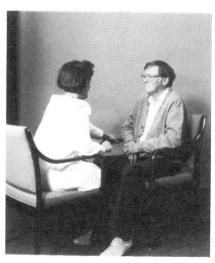

(Picture #8)

The caregiver is sitting directly in front, facing the client and leaning into the person. When the caregiver is asked why she is sitting in this manner, the response is usually, "I want to establish rapport." When questioned how that type of positioning can enhance rapport, the person will respond, "If I show the person I am not afraid of him, he will not be afraid of me." Wrong! That positioning and posture will only elevate anxiety for three reasons.

171

1) Leaning towards the client is intimidating. It is encroaching into the client's personal space. Due to recent memory loss, the client will not know who is in front of him. This will only result in elevating his anxiety level.

2) Sitting directly in front of the individual creates *forced eye contact*. In this position, the client is required to look directly at someone for an extended period of time. This requires concentration, attention span and high analytical ability. He is being pressured to function at a level that is beyond his ability. The longer this occurs, the higher his anxiety level.

3) Lastly, this face-to-face confrontation is confining. The client is virtually boxed into the chair. The only way he can leave is over top of the person in front of him.

This positioning often increases the client's anxiety level and contributes to an aggressive response.

SITTING TO THE SIDE

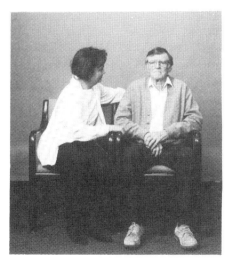

(Picture #9)

(Picture #9) This is probably one of the most common positions taken by many caregivers, and yet it creates the most obvious difficulty for the mentally impaired. Due to the loss of peripheral vision (the narrow or tunneled vision discussed in chapter one), and decreased flexibility to turn and look, the person sitting next to a mentally impaired client is out of the client's visual field. It may be possible to get the client's attention momentarily to ask a question, but when the client looks away he will not only forget the conversation, he will have lost awareness for the person sitting next to him.

CONTROLLING APPROACH

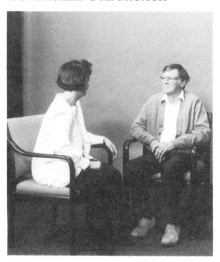

(Picture #10)

(Picture #10) Sitting at a right angle to the dominant side of a mentally impaired client is the most effective way to decrease anxiety, enhance rapport and maintain control. In this position, the caregiver is within the client's field of vision. (not intimidating by sitting in front of him or hiding from view by sitting to the side). Likewise, the caregiver is *inviting eye contact*, rather than forcing it. The client has the freedom to look at the caregiver as long as he is able, then look away when he feels pressured. Finally, if the client wants to leave he can simply stand up and go. There is no feeling of being confined or trapped.

This approach gives the client the feeling that he is in control. When that occurs, his anxiety remains at its tolerable level, and the potential for an aggressive response is minimized.

SUMMARY: SITTING WITH A CLIENT

If a client is right hand dominant, the following summary applies:

Controlling Approach	Cautions
1) Sit at right angles on the dominant side.	Do not sit in the front or to the side of the client.
2) Invite eye contact.	Do not force eye contact.

3) Allow the client the freedom to leave if he feels pressured.	Do not box him into the chair.

APPROACHING THE WALKING CLIENT FROM BEHIND

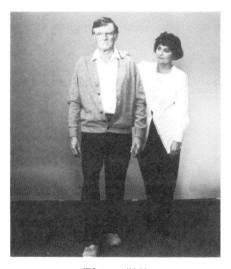

(Picture #11)

(Picture #11) Approaching a mentally impaired client from behind is best described as reality shock. The client has no warning of anyone being there. Suddenly he feels a hand on his shoulder. His anxiety will immediately elevate to a panic state and he will probably retaliate.

Take this one step further. It is common to watch caregivers come from behind a mentally impaired client to walk past him, without giving any warning of their presence. To encounter the suddenness of someone zipping past can be frightening. When one approaches a mentally impaired client from behind, it is best to give the person a wide birth and make a comment that you are coming around before he is reached. This at least provides warning of someone's presence, and an opportunity for the mentally impaired client to prepare as someone walks past.

APPROACHING THE WALKING CLIENT FROM THE FRONT

Approaching a mentally impaired client from the front creates the same dynamics that were demonstrated by sitting in a chair in front of the individual. (Picture #12).

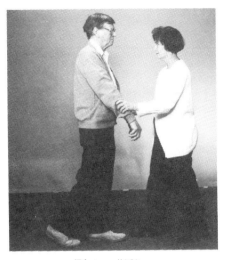
(Picture #12)

- Approaching from the front forces eye contact, elevating his anxiety level.
- The caregiver's posture encroaches into the client's space, and is intimidating.
- The client is restrained, he can no longer go forward.
- Abruptly stopping a mentally impaired client requires an immediate change in his thought process. He does not have the ability to adjust to the suddenness of the contact.
- The caregiver is not in control. She is unable to watch his two arms and legs. The chances of being struck or kicked are great.

THE CONTROLLING APPROACH

When approaching a mentally impaired client who he is walking, (Picture #13) there are a few strategies that will enhance rapport and assist the caregiver to be in control.

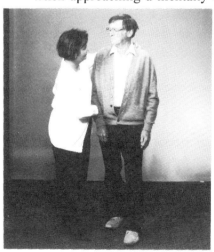
(Picture #13)

1) Approach at a right angle to the client, from his dominant side. In this way the caregiver is not intimidating or shocking him, but is in his field of vision. Likewise, standing to his side, prevents him from kicking.

2) Place your inside arm and hand on his shoulder. This light touch will enhance rapport. Remember to read his cueing. If he shrugs, it indicates of course that he does not want that contact, requiring the hand to be removed.

3) Notice that the caregiver's right hand is lightly against the client's right arm. Should the client attempt to strike, then the caregiver is able to control his movements. Do not grab his right wrist. If the client feels the caregiver grabbing him, he will react accordingly.

4) Gradually slow him down. Take an extra ten or so paces to allow his thought process to catch up with your actions.

SUMMARY: APPROACHING THE CLIENT WHO IS WALKING

If a client is right hand dominant, the following summary applies:

Controlling Approach	Cautions
1) Approach at a right angle on his dominant side.	Do not approach from the front or from the back.
2) Place the left arm over the shoulder of the client for rapport enhancement.	If the client shrugs or gives any indication that he is not comfortable, remove it.
3) Lightly place the right hand next to the client's right wrist.	Do not grab the client.
4) Continue ten or so paces forward, to slow the client to a stop.	Do not make the client come to an abrupt stop, it does not give him time to catch up with the caregiver's actions.

VOICE COMMAND

Giving verbal direction to a mentally impaired client when that person attempts to strike, pick up something that is dangerous or move into a situation that is unsafe, is always a valuable intervention. There are two factors that must be considered to make voice commands effective. They are voice tone and the command itself.

a) Voice Tone

We discussed earlier a hearing condition in aging called presbycusis. This causes an older client to lose the ability to hear high tones. It was demonstrated that caregivers with a lower voice tone may be better understood by certain mentally impaired clients than those with a higher voice tone.

When a caregiver becomes excited, nervous or surprised the natural response is to raise one voice's tone an octave or so higher when giving a verbal command such as - "Please don't do that." Or "Please don't go in there." As soon as the caregiver raises her voice an octave then comprehension by the mentally impaired client may be lost, and the client will probably not react in the manner that is desired.

Likewise, raising one's voice tone in such a situation will likely impede rapport. The suddenness of the caregiver's reaction, the inability to comprehend what is being said and the high pitched voice will only confuse the client further and potentially increase the person's agitation.

The objective of any approach is to enhance rapport and be in control. This does not mean that a caregiver has to talk in a baritone voice. However, it does require the caregiver to be conscious of controlling her voice tone. In situations where her or the client's safety is in jeopardy, then any verbal command must be given in the caregiver's normal voice tone. In this way comprehension may be increased and the client may respond in the manner required.

b) Command

There are often two problems with verbal commands given to a mentally impaired client during an aggressive response. Some caregivers employ something called verbiage - complex instructions or commands that bombard the client. Furthermore, there is often minimal consistency in the command given for specific actions or events. For example, when a client raises his arm to resist a caregiver while toileting, one caregiver may say - "John, you don't need to strike out at people when they attempt to help. If you would put your hand down it would make it easier." Another caregiver who experiences the same client action on the next occasion says in response, "John, please don't raise your hand like that. It is too hard to help you."

The problems with these two phrases are obvious. They provide for the client a verbal salad which he must digest before responding. His thought process will be unable to analyze the information quickly enough to react as requested.

Secondly, there may be consistency in the content of what the two caregivers are saying, but not in the words they are using. The mentally impaired experience this disparity as two different sets of instructions. Therefore the potential for comprehension is made even more difficult.

To be successful with the mentally impaired requires verbal instructions to be short and simple. In the example sighted above the response by both caregivers could be, "John, please stop," followed by lowering the client's hand. Whatever verbal command is found successful, it must be consistently utilized by all caregivers in contact with that client.

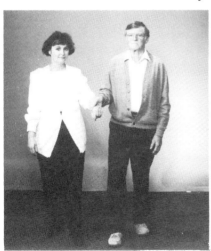

(Picture #14)

When the voice tone is controlled and the command is simple and short, then the possibility of comprehension by the mentally impaired is increased. In this way the caregiver may successfully defuse a potentially aggressive response.

WALKING WITH ASSISTANCE

Some clients will attempt to grab a caregiver's arm or hand as they walk down the hall. (Picture

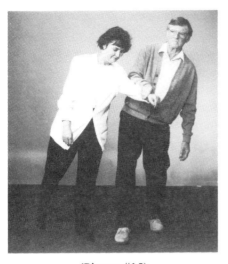

(Picture #15)

#14) This need to hold on is an attempt to compensate for the loss of balance.

The client requires the added support from the caregiver. The problem is that in this position, the caregiver is not in control. If something should occur that takes the client off guard, then the staff member will be feeling the client's nails in her arm.

More importantly, in this position the caregiver cannot provide adequate support. (picture #15) If the client should fall, the caregiver would be unable to react to pull the client back on balance. Leaving the potential for both to fall.

CONTROLLING APPROACH

(Picture #16) As soon as the client reaches for the caregiver's arm, she needs to reach back to the person's hand, open the grip by lifting

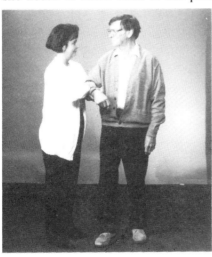

(Picture #16)

lightly on the palm. Then slide her left arm under the client's arm, placing her right hand on the client's forearm. This provides the greatest support, enhances rapport and ensures that the caregiver is in control.

If the client does fall, then the caregiver is able to use her weight and balance to pivot the client back. If the client wants to hold onto the caregiver's hand, she can slip the fingers of her left hand into the palm of the client's hand. If the client should be startled and begin to dig his nails into the caregiver's fingers, it is quite easy to pull them out of the client's grasp.

SUMMARY: APPROACHING THE CLIENT WHO IS WALKING

If a client is right hand dominant, the following summary applies:

Controlling Approach	Cautions
1) Approach the dominant side.	Do not approach the dominant side, the client has limited control.
2) When the client grabs the caregiver's arm, reach back to his hand and lightly open his grip by pulling up on the palm.	Make this a gentle motion. If the client has the feeling you are grabbing him, he will fight.
3) Slide your left arm under the client's elbow with the left arm, place the right hand on the client's forearm. Slip the fingers of the left hand into the client's hand.	Do not slip the right hand into the client's hand, it will be too difficult to draw it out.

APPROACHING A CLIENT WHO IS IN BED

In one case the caregiver stated that a client was more agitated when she was approached in bed than when approached in any other location. This is understandable.

Imagine:

> You are lying on your back in bed
> You are looking up/
> Two people approach you
> One on either side/
> When would you see them?
> Which one would you see first?

You would see them only when they were standing next to you, and you can only see one at a time. If you did not recognize these people, you would find yourself highly pressured, trying to look at one to determine who that person is, then look at the other.

For the mentally impaired, the experience is even more dramatic. The caregiver he would see first would be the one on her dominant side (a natural reflex response). Seeing that person would require him to invest considerable energy to determine who she is and what she wants. While this was occurring, he will only know that there is someone else present on his other side when that person touches him. There is no question that this would also be classified as reality shock. The suddenness of the contact will only initiate an aggressive response.

CONTROLLING APPROACH

When a caregiver approaches a mentally impaired client lying in bed, she must always approach from the dominate side. The client's reflex reaction will be to turn to the dominant side. If two staff are approaching the client in bed, the one on the non-dominant side must delay for a few seconds. The first caregiver on the client's dominant side approaches first. That caregiver then directs the client's attention to the approach of the other caregiver by saying something such as, "Mary has also come into see you Mr. Smith." In this way they have allowed his thought process to catch up with their actions and taken the necessary steps to prevent an aggressive response.

SUMMARY

Some are surprised at the investment of time and energy to describe these basic approaches to the mentally impaired. In actual fact, one of the most common causes for aggressive behavior of the mentally impaired is from an inappropriate approach. If those first few seconds of contact can enhance rapport and allow the caregiver to be on control, then the outcome will more than likely be positive

These past few chapters have uncovered the *investigative* caregiver's unique ability to perform what can be considered "magic" with the mentally impaired. This *magic* is the success with a certain mentally impaired client with whom others seem to be struggling. It is often the subtle differences that makes an investigative caregiver. Before moving to the last chapter, take time to compete the Programming Strategy Check List on the following page to uncover how much of the material presented in these past chapters you can recall.

PROGRAM STRATEGY CHECKLIST

When you decided to read this text, I guarantee that it was not merely to pass the time. You wanted to gain more information about Alzheimer's aggression and ways to deal with it effectively. Like most of us, you probably did not have the opportunity to read this book from start to finish all at once. You undoubtedly read a section, put the book down and then returned to it when the opportunity presented itself.

This text has provided a number of strategies that are valuable in preventing Alzheimer's aggression. *Take the time* to review the following checklist of assessment and programming options to see how well you can recall what was discussed. If the strategy is well understood, then check in the column marked "*Clear.*" If you cannot easily recall the strategy and its purpose, then mark the column identified as "*Review.*" A reference page number has been provided that will allow you a quick reference to the section detailing that section.

Assessment	*Clear*	*Review*
Precursors To Aggressive Behavior (page 194) A measuring tool that defines the working environment and how it may contribute to the aggressive response of the mentally impaired.		
Client Profile (page 114) This summary overview, or client profile, provides a detailed assessment that will often uncover secrets, patterns, relationship of behaviors, response to schedules and events, etc.		
Patterning (page 107) There are two components to patterning - the time pattern and the event pattern. These will identify the intervention strategies needed to decrease or eliminate the distresser.		

	Clear	Review
Pre-emptive Cueing (page 106) Defining the signals that indicates when a mentally impaired client is distressed.		
Care Analysis (page 111) Care analysis is a problem identification mechanism utilized during the care conference. It allows all members of the care team to brainstorm what may be causing a client's behavior or change in functioning		
Comprehension board (page 128) This tool is used to define verbal, task and performance comprehension.		
Aggressive Profile (page 121) Defining: Who has less of a problem or no problem? Who has the most difficulty with this client?		
Aggressive Episodes (page 131) Each aggressive episode, regardless of its severity, must be examined thoroughly by a series of analysis questions.		
Progressive Functioning (page 126) Involves determining how long it takes the person's thought process to catch up with the actions of others.		
Diversional Tactics (page 117) Attempting to uncover what will illicit negative emotions and what thought process will capture positive emotions.		
Interview (page 123) Intended to define: attention span, emotional state, language pattern, thought process, reminiscing ability		

	Clear	Review
Recreational Programming (page 130) The initial assessment of activities is to determine the programming opportunities that exist for the mentally impaired of varying abilities.		
Dosage & Dispensing Pattern (page 110) Used to define specific patterns of behavior in order to discover causative factors and alternate intervention strategies.		
Client Log (page 118) Placed at the front of the chart, staff are then instructed to record anything they discover about this client from any source (other than confidential information).		
Past History (page 119) Specific questions that family must be asked to understand a client's aggressive behavior. Attempting to define the relationship between past events and personality qualities to present behavior.		
Live on the Unit (page 130) Organizational representatives are responsible to do a thorough analysis of the pressures encountered by the mentally impaired on that unit.		
Intuition (page 131) Based on two solid pieces of information: *Experience and Knowing the Person.*		

	Clear	Review
PROGRAMMING		
Retracting (page 143) These strategies remove the distresser and leave the client alone to settle.		

	Clear	Review
Diverting (page 148) These are strategies employed during times of distress intended to change the clients emotional state by changing the individual's thought process.		
Redirecting (page 152) These tactics remove the individual from the distresser and focus the client's energy elsewhere.		
Chaotic Events (page 143) After a chaotic event all programming will be delayed for one hour for some mentally impaired clients. Others will require all but basic care stopped for the remainder of the day.		
Unit Monitor (page 146) The responsibility of the Unit Monitor is to determine the appropriateness of what is to occur, given what is happening on the unit at that time.		
Energy Conservation (page 148) Rest or nap periods remove a mentally impaired client from the accumulation of stressors, decreases anxiety, and provides the individual the opportunity to recharge physical and mental energies in preparation for the next barrage of stimuli.		
Family (page 149) The presence of family commonly has associated with it positive past memories. In many instances a mentally impaired client will soon forget what was distressing and smile at the presence of a family member.		

	Clear	Review
Cue words (page 150) These are words that will *immediately* snap a mentally impaired client into past positive memory, changing emotional state and changing behavior.		
Topics of Conversation (page 151) Focusing on certain topics and expanding them will often draw a mentally impaired client back into a past memory. The more the person recalls that memory, the more a change in her emotional state and behavior will be noticed.		
Pictures of Keepsake Items (page 151) May draw the client back to a past positive thought process and elicit a positive emotional response to counter the distresser experienced.		
Music (page 151) "Old fashioned music" is often an effective distracter for many mentally impaired clients, whether through a sing-a-long, record player or radio.		
Sensory Stimulation (page 152) These tools are used to stimulate the senses - touch, smell, sight and/or taste and are used to subsequently recall past events. (specifically Theme Boxes)		
Chores (page 153) Activities such as cleaning table tops, assisting with laundry, sweeping, etc. do not have to be learned. They relate well to the individual's past history.		

	Clear	Review
Walking (page 153) The goal of a walking program for certain mentally impaired clients during times of distress is to identify the furthest and fastest the person can safely go.		
Relaxation Techniques (page 153) These are employed formally and informally with the mentally impaired - back or foot massage, hot baths, deep breathing exercises (if the client is able to follow direction).		
Drug Utilization Strategies (page 154) Proactive use of medication to assist the client over the worst time of the day when no other programming options are available.		

CONTROLLING APPROACH	Clear	Review
Approaching The Client Who is Sitting (page 162) 1. Approach from the right side. 2. Move any chair or obstacle away from the client's right side. 3. Crouch down below eye level. 4. Place the left hand lightly on the client's right wrist, the right elbow lightly on the client's right knee, right leg against the clients right leg. 5. Keep your body away from the client		
Sitting With A Client (page 173) 1. Sit at right angles on the dominant side. 2. Invite eye contact. 3. Allow the client the freedom to leave if he feels pressured.		

	Clear	Review
Approaching The Walking Client (page 175) 1. Approach at a right angle on his dominant side. 2. Place the left arm over the shoulder of the client for rapport enhancement. 3. Lightly place the right hand next to the client's right wrist. 4. Continue ten or so paces forward, to slow the client to a stop.		
Walking with Assistance (page 179) 1. Approach the dominant side. 2. When the client grabs the caregiver's arm, reach back to his hand and lightly open his grip by pulling up on the palm. 3. Slide your left arm under the client's elbow with the left arm, place the right hand on the client's forearm. Slip the fingers of the left hand into the client's hand.		
Approaching The Client in Bed (page 181) 1. Caregiver on the client's dominant side approaches first. 2. Then directs the client's attention to the approach of the other caregiver.		
Step Process Approach (page 171) The approach begins four feet from the client. The goal is to seek eye contact before moving closer. This can be accomplished by calling the client's name.		
Voice Command (page 177) In situations where the caregiver or client's safety is in jeopardy, then any verbal command must be given in the caregiver's normal voice tone. Verbal instructions must be short, simple and consistently used by all caregivers.		

Chapter Eight

MEETING THE CHALLENGE

There has been a constant theme throughout this text .

> It was never -   How do we change the mentally
> impaired.

> Instead it was - *How do we change for the mentally
> impaired.*

There is such a diverse response to the material presented. Some organizations already do much of what was discussed, and excel to the next level of care. The majority of organizations are striving to achieve a conducive care environment for this clientele, and find this material appropriate. Yet there are others who will exclaim that the philosophy and material presented in this text is totally unrealistic. This diversity in responses is nothing new.

Long term care in the late sixties and early seventies exhibited the same contradictions when discussing care for the cognitively well, physically disabled older client. In those early days, the industry provided basic care.

> ⇒   Bed sores were a common occurrence in many organization. They were so severe at times, that they were actual holes to the bone.
> ⇒   Bedridden clients were in a frozen fetal position due to flexion contractures. Once they reached a certain state of dependency, little was done with them other then the most basic of care.
> ⇒   The physical environment was stark and sterile, with little personalization and minimal emphasis on a home-like character.

⇒ Medication use for any behavior that challenged the care routine was substantial.

⇒ Rules and routines were highly structured. Staff were primarily technicians, being told what was to be done each day, and given little freedom to vary.

⇒ The opportunity for formal training was limited. The industry itself was not seen as a specialty. Education for direct line staff was minimal.

⇒ The success of recreational programs was measured not by the individual's response, but by the number of clients who attended the program, willingly or otherwise.

⇒ There was limited individuality in care. The care environment was quite homogenous.

⇒ Care planning, assessment tools, programming, if they did exist, were often quite basic.

Generally, custodial care was the norm, quality of care was the exception. When challenged, many organizations agreed with the need to change, but they always presented the same excuses that prevented that change from occurring - never enough money, resources or staff.

Yet there were the exceptions and they were impressive. These were organizations who refused to except the norm of the day. They were highly creative groups of professionals determined to make the situation for the cognitively well elderly *different*. Working with the same money, resources and staffing as the rest, they dramatically improved the living environment for the frail elderly. They created individualized, quality programming conducive to the needs of the physically disabled. They proved that it could be done.

What was interesting was the response to their accomplishments. Some organizations followed their lead. They intentionally moved along, changing as they could, using the leaders within the industry to direct them on how to enhance the care they performed. Other organizations on the other hand saw these "leaders" as the exceptions. They believed that what went on in the progressive organizations did not realistically apply to their own setting. They always perceived the leaders as having more money, staff, and resources, or that their circumstances were different, or that . . . The organizations satisfied with the status quo did not believe that their own staff had the ability or desire to perform in the creative manner demonstrated by the leaders. Therefore, they were unwilling to invest the energy and time to develop their people and their environment to enhance the quality. They simply dragged their feet, believing that what they did was "good enough."

Soon the example of the leaders and the efforts of the majority of organizations changed the industry standards as a whole. The goal within long term care became quality, individualized care. Those who were reluctant to follow were virtually pushed into action through peer pressure and legislation. Today there are few organizations that do not have a resident council, care plans, monitoring of chemical and physical restraints, re-activation programming, home-like and personalized environments, etc. Generally, our industry cares well for the cognitively well, physically disabled client.

Now our industry faces a new challenge - the mentally impaired elderly. Most long term care facilities have a client population of 50-60% who demonstrate a measurable degree of mental impairment. That percentage will only increase over time. It will soon be possible that there will not be a need for a specialized unit for the mentally impaired. Instead many long term care facilities will require a specialized unit for the cognitively well, physically disabled, given that their numbers will be so limited in comparison to the mentally impaired.

Long term care, both institutional and community based, are at a similar transition point now as in the past. There are organizations that are doing an excellent job with the mentally impaired. They have empowered their staff to take ownership, instilled flexibility within the care routine, provided their caregivers with the needed training, and an array of tools and supports to adapt to the mentally impaired. Yet, there are those who have not changed.

The old system no longer works. The needs of the mentally impaired are dramatically different than the needs of the cognitively well. However, the outcome, if those needs are not met, is different as well.

When discussing the do's and don'ts in caring for the mentally impaired, the focus is not only on quality of life for the individual client. It is also on the efficiency and effectiveness of the organization, as well as the safety of its staff. If effective programming is not defined and enforced, and the care environment adapted to meet the needs of this clientele, then the mentally impaired will simply exhaust the organization's resources. What will result will be an:

⇒ *increase* in aggressive behavior.
⇒ *increase* in medication use.
⇒ *increase* in dependency.
⇒ *increase* in work load.
⇒ *decrease* in staff morale.
⇒ *increase* in sick time.
⇒ *increase* in staff demand.
⇒ *increase* in violent behavior.
⇒ *increase* in staff injuries.

Do I need to go on? This clientele does not allow us the luxury of time to adapt. Their needs are immediate. The incidence of aggressive behavior of the mentally impaired is totally related to the care environment in which this person lives.

If the care environment is specific to meet the needs of the mentally impaired, aggressive/violent episodes will be minimal.

If the care environment is not specific to meet the needs of the mentally impaired, aggressive/violent episodes will be substantial.

To prevent Alzheimer's aggression effectively, the focus must be on the care environment. Given the diversity in the organizations caring for this clientele, each has a different need.

Those organizations who excel in caring for the mentally impaired are challenged to enhance what they are already doing. Those organizations are the ground breakers, the pacesetters for the industry. For them, this text not only provides skills that they may adapt into their care routine, but *reinforces* what they ascribe.

To those organizations who are striving to reach this pentacle of care, the need is different. The material presented in this text is intended to provide a clearer understanding of the need and effective strategies that can be employed to prevent aggression. The goal is to *motivate* them to take the next step and provide clarity on what needs to be addressed.

To those working in organizations where the needs of this clientele are still not met and programming is at its infancy, the expectations must be different. This text has attempted to demonstrate the urgency, and to provide you the *confidence* to challenge your workplace to actively define the care environment as it applies to the mentally impaired.

Before programming is examined, much of the work to decrease aggressive behavior focuses on the care environment in which this person lives and the caregiver's doing the care.

THE PRECURSORS TO AGGRESSIVE BEHAVIOR

It is difficult to prevent Alzheimer's aggression if the care environment in which that person lives is not supportive of programming needs. Complete the following questionnaire based on your work setting:

How consistent is care?

1------2------3-----4-----5
minimal   very

How knowledgeable are those doing the care:

about the disease?

1------2------3-----4-----5
minimal   very

about the specialized programming and care strategies?

1------2------3-----4-----5
minimal   very

about assessment techniques?

1------2------3-----4-----5
minimal   very

How flexible are:

staff?

1------2------3-----4-----5
minimal   very

managers?

1------2------3-----4-----5
minimal   very

routines?   1------2------3-----4-----5
                                 minimal   very

How demanding is   1------2------3-----4-----5
    the care routine?   minimal   very

How effective is the communication process:

    between shifts?   1------2------3-----4-----5
                                 minimal   very

    between departments?   1------2------3-----4-----5
                                 minimal   very

    between   1------2------3-----4-----5
    staff/management?   minimal   very

    with family?   1------2------3-----4-----5
                                 minimal   very

How tolerable are staff to a   1------2------3-----4-----5
    client's resistive behavior?   minimal   very

How objective are staff towards 1------2------3-----4-----5
    aggressive/violent   minimal   very
    behavior?

How effective is the care team at 1------2------3-----4-----5
    problem solving   minimal   very
    client behavior?

How involved are the direct care staff in decision making:

    about care?   1------2------3-----4-----5
                                 minimal   very

    about the unit?   1------2------3-----4-----5
                                 minimal   very

How disruptive is the environment:

noise level?	1------2------3-----4-----5
	very minimal
clutter/crowded?	1------2------3-----4-----5
	very minimal
activity level?	1------2------3-----4-----5
	very minimal

Add the numbers allocated to each question for a **Total Score** _____

The mentally impaired themselves become the barometers to measure the effectiveness of an organization in consistency, communication, problem solving, etc. If the scoring to this questionnaire totals below 60 the chances are high that aggressive behavior is common place and the usage of chemical and/or physical restraints are high. A scoring above 85 will often uncover a minimal use of chemical and/or physical restraints, and little aggressive/violent behavior.

Do not let the total score be the only indicator of need. The answer to each question plays a significant role in programming success. An organization can have a high overall score except for one or two areas. It is this that can impact on the client's behavior and must be addressed.

Use this questionnaire in your workplace to identify what may be blocking effective care. (A copy of this questionnaire for photocopying is located in the addendum, page 209.) Provide a copy of the questionnaire to a cross section of both staff and managers. Ask them not to sign their copy. However, request that staff place an "S" at the top of their copy, and managers place an "M" at the top of theirs.

Gather the completed copies and tally the results. Add the accumulative total to each question for staff and managers separately. For example, if thirty staff score a total of 96 points for the first question, then the staff average is (96 divided by 30) 3.2 for that question. If sixteen managers score a total of 38 points for the same question, then their average response for that question is (38 divided by

16) 2.4. Then compare how the staff see the care environment with how the managers see it.

    ⇒ If both staff and managers score high on a certain question, then it is a strength and supports programming effectiveness.

    ⇒ If both staff and managers score low on a certain question, then that issue must be resolved in order to prevent aggression.

    ⇒ If staff score low and managers high on the same question, then this can be interpreted in many different ways. Primarily it reflects that the expectation of managers may not be fully achieved, requiring the situation to be investigated in order for it to be resolved.

    ⇒ If managers score low and staff score high, again there can be different interpretations. Primarily, it reflects that the managers have not fully communicated their expectations, and must demonstrate to staff the limitations experienced, and gain their motivation to resolve it.

When these issues are addressed, the potential for preventing Alzheimer's aggression is very real.

CAREGIVER

Knowing that there is no formula, no cook book to effectively care for the mentally impaired, places the greatest challenge on the caregiver. When assessing aggressive/violent episodes, one of the components of that assessment is to investigate who was on duty the eight to sixteen hours before the incident occurred. In an environment where staff are not consistent, programming is not defined or enforced, caregivers are not trained, the pressure on the client can be intense.

There are two issues that may explain the limited tolerance of some caregivers to certain behaviors - personal experiences and expectations of the client.

Personal Experiences - There are caregivers who have had very negative experiences with aggression in their personal history. These are individuals who are oversensitive to the behaviors of others. This may be due to their being dominated by aggression throughout their life, even to the extreme of abuse. When any aggressive behavior is encountered now, those past experiences are recalled. This results in the caregiver personalizing the situation and losing their objectivity.

Other caregivers have had no experience with aggression, either personally or professionally. They have not learned how to cope with it. When encountered, they become highly fearful and overreact to the slightest elevation of a client's mood.

Each of these caregivers requires assistance in depersonalizing the client's behavior in order to maintain their objectivity. They require:

⇒ formal education.
⇒ buddying with staff who are comfortable with aggressive behavior who can assist them when the behavior is encountered.
⇒ counseling through an employee assistance program.

Expectations of the Client - Other caregivers who have difficulty with aggressive behavior are those who are strong nurturers. These are individuals who seem to easily personalize the client's behavior as though it were a reflection on the "care" they provide. They read the client's behavior as though it were a criticism of their performance. Their intolerance is often based on a dictum of "shoulds." - the client:

should understand that the caregiver is trying to help.
should understand the importance of what is being done.
should remember the last time the care was done.
should be cooperative.
should be able to adapt.
should know how difficult he is making it.

should know that other people are in need as well.
should know that the caregiver is busy.

Even though these caregivers will admit that the client has lost recent memory and analytical ability, they never seem to apply that to their personal dealings with the client. These caregivers lack the needed flexibility. They assume that the client understands who they are, what they are doing, and why. Needless to say, that comprehension and recall is impossible for the mentally impaired.

Formal education in understanding the clientele and the premise for programming would be of value. More significantly, it seems that these caregivers need specific direction on how to be flexible with each case, and then held accountable should they not comply.

SELF ASSESSMENT

The questionnaire "Precursors to Aggressive Behavior" evaluated your work environment. Complete the following questionnaire to evaluate how well you perform in your care of the mentally impaired. Be honest, no one will look at your response. The goal is to define what is needed for you to enhance your own ability in this area.

How much do I ensure that what
is done by the care team
is consistent?

1------2------3-----4-----5
minimal   very

How knowledgeable am I:

about the disease?

1------2------3-----4-----5
minimal   very

about the specialized
programming and care
strategies?

1------2------3-----4-----5
minimal   very

about assessment
techniques?

1------2------3-----4-----5
minimal   very

How tolerable am I
    to a client's resistive
    behavior?

1------2------3-----4-----5
minimal   very

How comfortable am I with
    aggressive/violent
    behavior?

1------2------3-----4-----5
minimal   very

How effective is am I at
    problem solving
    client behavior?

1------2------3-----4-----5
minimal   very

How flexible am I in what I do?

1------2------3-----4-----5
minimal   very

How well do I communicate:

    to other caregivers?

1------2------3-----4-----5
minimal   very

    to other departments?

1------2------3-----4-----5
minimal   very

    to families?

1------2------3-----4-----5
minimal   very

As staff, how involved am I in decision making/
As a manager, how much do I involve staff
    in the decision making?

    about care?

1------2------3-----4-----5
minimal   very

    about the unit?

1------2------3-----4-----5
minimal   very

Add the numbers allocated to each question for a **Total Score** _____

Use this questionnaire within your organization as well. (A copy is available for photocopying in the addendum, page 211). When staff and managers complete the assessment about the organization, have them complete this self assessment as well. Tabulate the scores to see whether there is disparity between how the staff and managers see themselves versus others.

> If the average scores for each question in the self assessment matches the same average scores for the organization assessment, then the chances for all to cooperate in developing programming for the mentally impaired is high. Generally staff and managers see how their personal performance contributes to programming needs. Admitting the need is the first step to program development.

> If the average scores for each question in the self assessment is higher than the average score for the organization assessment, then you will have a greater challenge. The belief by staff and managers is that their individual performance does not contribute to the need. These individuals may require more personal direction to understand their role in meeting programming objectives.

WHAT DO _YOU_ STAND FOR

I have had the pleasure of presenting seminars to thousands of caregivers over the years. It is invigorating to witness how excited participants become about the material presented. They nod their heads in agreement that what is professed matches the philosophy that they themselves hold for the mentally impaired.

Yet when some of those individuals return to their workplace, it seems that things change. When they encounter limited resources, other staff who do not agree and/or mangers who are not supportive, they abandon their philosophy. They tend to take the easier course and maintain the status quo which contradicts everything they profess. A question for you:

How much power do you give others to influence
who you are and
what you do?

It is easy to profess what you believe in. Yet you never really know what you stand for until you are challenged. There is nothing that I admire more than watching individuals in the seminar become excited, agree with the philosophy, return to their workplace, and no matter what they encounter, they are determined to maintain what they profess.

"They walk the talk."

The material in this text has everything to do with the mentally impaired and nothing to do with the mentally impaired. Although the content describes the disease process and the vulnerability, in actual fact there is nothing that the mentally impaired can do differently then what they are doing. They are locked in a disease that has for them no way out. The quality of their life is not dependent on their actions, but on yours.

This text has been about **you**. What **you** do. What **you** profess. What **you** believe in. The mentally impaired need leaders - those willing to be their advocates, who will defend their individuality. Individuals who are not satisfied with the status quo, but are willing to meet the challenges. The *investigative caregivers* are those leaders - are **you**?

ADDENDUM

You have permission to photocopy:

The Client Profile

to be used as an assessment tool for the mentally impaired elderly clients under the care of your organization __only__.

You have permission to photocopy the following questionnaires to be distributed to the staff and managers of your organization __only__.

1) Precursors to Aggressive Behavior
2) Self Assessment

Conditions for use include the following:

1) The copyright must remain with any copy.
2) The documents are not to be used outside of your organization.
3) You are free to adapt these documents as long as any changes are communicated to the author.

Any other use or duplication in part or in whole other than specified above without permission in writing by the author.

CLIENT PROFILE

The questionnaire is to be initiated by a caregiver who best knows the client in question. The completed questionnaire is then reviewed by each shift (days, afternoons and nights).

Past History - what do you know about this individual regarding: family, work, accomplishments, likes/dislikes, leisure activities, etc.

Personality Characteristics - Identify what you know about this person regarding self image (dress and appearance), how this person dealt with stress in the past, dependency on others, rituals, dominant personality qualities, etc.

The next sections deal with what the person is experiencing now.

PRESENT STATE

What behaviors or symptoms does this person demonstrate?	When do they occur? (if known)

Present Drug Regime

Drug Ordered	Dosage/ Frequency	Reason Ordered	Date Order Began

Past Drug Regime

Drug Ordered	Dosage/ Frequency	Reason Ordered	Date Began	Date Stop

*If PRN **sedation** is being used - look for any time pattern when they are dispensed.*

PRN Sedation	Dosage	Time Pattern

Daily Profile - Outline this individual's normal day, identifying hour by hour activities of daily living, how time is spent, recreational activities, etc. Define what this person does in detail and the individual's response to each event. Add at the bottom anything done weekly or monthly, i.e. bath or certain recreational activities, etc.

Time	Activity	Response

POINT OF CHANGE

Identify a time in the recent past where this person looked, acted or performed differently then what would be seen today. Describe that person back then, including behavior, abilities, care needs, etc. that would not be seen today.

When is this person's "worse time" of the day?

How will the person respond (behavior, refusal/inability to perform tasks) during that time?

What usually occurs around or to the client during and after that time?

What is required to settle the individual? What will be the result (behavior, refusal/inability to perform tasks)? How long before he/she will return to "his/her normal self?"

ENHANCING FUNCTIONING ABILITY

What needs to be told to a "new" caregiver about this client that will allow that person to be successful?

What would you like to see different about this client than what is being done now? (regarding care, activities, medication, treatment, etc.)

THE PRECURSORS TO AGGRESSIVE BEHAVIOR

Complete the following questionnaire based on your work setting. Do not sign your copy. Staff are asked to place an "S" at the top of their copy, and managers to place an "M" at the top of theirs.

How consistent is care?

1------2------3-----4-----5
minimal   very

How knowledgeable are those doing the care:

about the disease?

1------2------3-----4-----5
minimal   very

about the specialized programming and care strategies?

1------2------3-----4-----5
minimal   very

about assessment techniques?

1------2------3-----4-----5
minimal   very

How flexible are:

staff?

1------2------3-----4-----5
minimal   very

managers?

1------2------3-----4-----5
minimal   very

routines?

1------2------3-----4-----5
minimal   very

How demanding is
the care routine?

1------2------3-----4-----5
minimal   very

How effective is the communication process:

between shifts?

1------2------3-----4-----5
minimal   very

between departments?

1------2------3-----4-----5
minimal   very

between staff/management?	1------2------3-----4-----5 minimal very
with family?	1------2------3-----4-----5 minimal very
How tolerable are staff to a client's resistive behavior?	1------2------3-----4-----5 minimal very
How objective are staff towards aggressive/violent behavior?	1------2------3-----4-----5 minimal very
How effective is the care team at problem solving client behavior?	1------2------3-----4-----5 minimal very

How involved are the direct care staff in decision making:

about care?	1------2------3-----4-----5 minimal very
about the unit?	1------2------3-----4-----5 minimal very

How disruptive is the environment:

noise level?	1------2------3-----4-----5 very minimal
clutter/crowded?	1------2------3-----4-----5 very minimal
activity level?	1------2------3-----4-----5 very minimal

Add the numbers allocated to each question for a **Total Score** _____

SELF ASSESSMENT

Complete the following questionnaire to evaluate how well you perform in caring for the mentally impaired. Do not sign your copy. Staff are asked to place an "S" at the top of their copy, and managers to place an "M" at the top of theirs.

How much do I ensure that what is done by the care team is consistent?

1------2------3-----4-----5
minimal   very

How knowledgeable am I:

about the disease?

1------2------3-----4-----5
minimal   very

about the specialized programming and care strategies?

1------2------3-----4-----5
minimal   very

about assessment techniques?

1------2------3-----4-----5
minimal   very

How tolerable am I

to a client's resistive behavior?

1------2------3-----4-----5
minimal   very

How comfortable am I with aggressive/violent behavior?

1------2------3-----4-----5
minimal   very

How effective is the care team at problem solving client behavior?

1------2------3-----4-----5
minimal   very

How flexible am I in what I do?

1------2------3-----4-----5
minimal   very

How well do I communicate:

      to other caregivers?   1------2------3-----4-----5
                                                   minimal   very

      to other departments?   1------2------3-----4-----5
                                                     minimal   very

      to families?   1------2------3-----4-----5
                                                     minimal   very

As staff how involved am I in decision making/
     As a manager how much do I involve staff
          in the decision making?

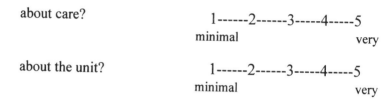

      about care?   1------2------3-----4-----5
                                                     minimal   very

      about the unit?   1------2------3-----4-----5
                                                  minimal   very

Add the numbers allocated to each question for a **Total Score** _____

BIBLIOGRAPHY

Asken, Michael J., Hartlage, Lawrence C. and Hornsby, J. Larry; *Essentials of Neuropsychological Assessment*; Springer Publishing Company Inc.; 1987

Bayly, Rich and Larue, Gerald A.; *Long-Term Care In an Aging Society: Choices and Challenges for the '90's*; Prometheus Books; 1992

Brodie, H. Keith H. and Houpt, Jeffrey L.; *Consultation-Liaison Psychiatry and Behavioral Medicine*; J.B. Lippincott Company; 1986

Cohen, Donna and Eisdorfer, Carl; *The Loss of Self: A Family Resource For The Care Of Alzheimer's Disease and Related Disorders*; W. W. Norton & Company; 1986

Cohen. Gene; *The Brain in Human Aging*; Springer Publishing Company Inc.; 1988

Corby, Nancy H., Downing, Richard, Lindeman, David A., and Sanborn, Beverly; *Alzheimer's Day Care: A Basic Guide*; Hemisphere Publishing Corp.; 1991

Deutsch, Georg and Springer, Sally P.; *Left Brain Right Brain*; W.H. Freeman and Company; 1981

Down, Ivy M. and Schnurr, Lorraine, *Between Home and Nursing Home; Prometheus Books*; 1991

Fabiano, Len; *Getting Staff Excited: The Nurse Manager (& Others Too) in Long Term Care; (second edition)*; FCS Publications; 1995

Fabiano, Len; *Mother I'm Doing The Best I Can*: *The Families of Aging Parents During Times of Loss and Crisis*; FCS Publications; 1991

Fabiano, Len; *The Tactics of Supportive Therapy: A Comprehensive Intervention Program For Effective Caring of the Alzheimer's Victim (second edition)*; FCS Publications;1993

Fabiano, Len; *Working withThe Frail Elderly: Beyond The Physical Disability*; FCS Publications;1989

Ferri, Richard S.; *Care Planning for the Older Adult: Nursing Diagnosis in Long Term Care*; W. B. Saunders Company; 1994

Flach, Frederic; *Affective Disorders*; The Hatherleigh Co. Ltd.; 1988

Gazzaniga, Michael S.; *Mind Matters: How The Mind & Brain Interact To Create Our Conscious Lives*; Houghton Mifflin Company; 1988

Grave, David J., Panzer, B.I.; *Resolving Traumatic Memories*; Irvington Publishers Inc.; 1991

Gruetzner, Howard; *Alzheimer's: A Caregiver's Guide and Sourcebook*; John Wiley & Sons Inc.; 1992

Gwyther, Lisa P.; *Care of Alzheimer's Patients; a Manual for Nursing Home Staff*; American Health Care Association; 1985

Harris, Grant T., Rice, Marnie E., Quinsey, Vernon L., Varney, George W.; *Violence in Institutions*: Understanding, Prevention and Control; Hans Huber Publishers Inc.; 1989

Jarvik, Lissy F. and Winograd, Carol Hutner; *Treatments for the Alzheimer Patient*; Springer Publishing Company Inc.; 1988

Kahn, Sherry and Saulo, Mileva; *Healing Yourself: A Nurse's Guide to Self-Care and Renewal*; Delmar Publishers Inc.; 1994

Kandel Hyman, Helen and Silverston, Barbara; *You and Your Aging Parent: A Family Guide to Emotional, Physical, and Financial Problems*; Random House of Canada Ltd.; 1989

Kociol, Lori and Schiff, Myra; *Alzheimers: A Canadian Family Resource Guide*; McGraw-Hill Ryerson Ltd.; 1989

Koff, Theodore H.; *New Approaches To Health Care For An Aging Population*; Jossey-Bass Inc; 1988

Leszcz, Molyn and Sadavoy, Joel; *Treating the Elderly With Psychotherapy: The Scope for Change in Later Life*; International Universities Press Inc.; 1987

McPherson, Barry D.; *Aging as a Social Process: An Introduction to Individual and Population Aging*; Butterworths Canada Ltd.; 1990

Ornstein, Robert and Thompson, Richard F.; The *Amazing Brain*; Houghton Mifflin Company; 1984

Polgar, Alex T., Singer, Carolyn and Wells, Lilian M.; *To Enhance Quality of Life In Institutions*; Canadian Scholars Press; 1992

Powell, Lenore S.; *Alzheimer's Disease: A Guide for Families*; Addison-Wesley Publishing Company; 1993

Pritchard, Jacki; *The Abuse of Elderly People: A Handbook for Professionals*; Jessica Kingsley Publishers Ltd.; 1992

Rhodes, Ann; *The Eldercare Sourcebook*; Key Porter Books Ltd.; 1993

Ross, Marvin; *The Silent Epidemic; A Comprehensive Guide To Alzheimer's Disease*; Hounslow Press; 1987

Rotenberg , Gerald N.; *Compendium of Pharmaceuticals and Specialties*; Canadian Pharmaceutical Association; 1995

Spratto, George R. and Woods, Adrienne L.; *NDR-92 Nurse's Drug Reference*; Delmar Publishers Inc.; 1992

Stern, E. Mark; *Psychotherapy and the Abrasive Patient*; The Haworth Press Inc.; 1984

Warren, Tom; *Beating Alzheimer's: A Step Towards Unlocking The Mysteries of Brain Diseases*; Tom Warren; 1991

INDEX

functioning, 103

quality care
    focus, 78, 98
    setting, 82
quality of life, 135

race, 89
rapport, 10, 11
rapport enhancement, 160, 165, 167, 176, 189
reality conflict, 19
rebound effect, 66
recent memory, 6, 7, 12, 20
recreation staff, 142
recreational
    activities, 151
    programming, 130
re-direct, 138, 142
redirecting, 152
reflex, 163
relaxation techniques, 153, 154
reminiscing ability, 103
repetitive speech, 137
resistive response, 75
resolve, 52
restoril, 47
restraint, 43
retracting, 143, 148
rummaging & hoarding, 22

secondary
    factors, 26, 54-58
    language loss, 86
secrets, 105, 106, 114
self assessment, 199
senile
    dementia of the alzheimer's type, 14
    plaques, 15